Making Anatomy and Physiology Easy

Tiffany Shepley James, B.S., M.S.

I would like to dedicate this book to

Vaughn C. Shepley, a hero among heroes.

This book was totally inspired by the love of my life, Alan James and my two little girls. I love you more than you will ever fathom.

I would also like to thank Allan and Lisa Shepley for the life-long support of my passion for science. I love you!

Table of Contents

CHAPTER 1

Oh NO! Not the cell AGAIN!

Ummm…yes. How do you expect to understand anything physiological if you don't remember anything from your introduction to general biology course? If we don't understand the cell at its base level we can never hope to understand anything about physiology. *WAIT!!! You don't remember what physiology means?!* Well let's clear that up right now.

Here's the fancy definition:

> Physiology: a branch of biological science that describes the functions of life or of living matter (as organs, tissues, or cells) and of the physical and chemical processes involved.

What that really means in plain English:

> Physiology: how stuff works.

Wow, now isn't that much easier to understand? Anatomy is the study of internal and external body structures and their relationship with other body parts. More simply said, how the parts look and how they are connected with other parts. Physiology is understanding how those parts work.

So back to the cell...

Let's take a look at the chalkboard…

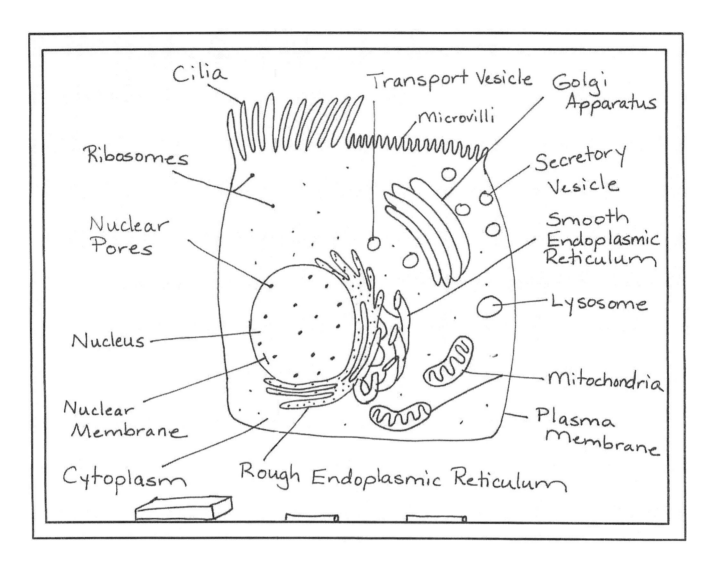

Okay so isn't it pretty? Sure, but how in the world am I going to remember all of those tiny parts? Those tiny parts are called <u>organelles</u>. Hopefully, you remember from your intro biology course that organelles are made of <u>molecules</u>, which are made of <u>atoms</u>. Whoa that's small!

Organelles are "tiny organs" that make up the cell and play important roles to help the cell survive—just like your organs help you to survive! An approach that helped me most is to imagine the cell is a city. Yes, a city. Work with me.

<u>Nucleus</u>—usually the largest organelle in the cell. It's the genetic control center (remember this is where the DNA is kept), and directs protein production in the cell. (These are pretty important jobs—sounds like this guy is in charge. We'll call this the governing body of the cell city)

<u>Plasma Membrane</u>—keeps what's out of the cell out and what's in the cell in. It will also allow communication between cells. It is made up of a phospholipid bilayer. (These are the cell city gates)

Ribosome—small granules that read the DNA and make protein. (Part of manufacturing plant of cell city)

Rough Endoplasmic Reticulum—collection of membranes studded with ribosomes which make it look rough like sandpaper. The rough ER helps make protein that is shipped out in transport vesicles. (Part of the manufacturing plant of cell city)

Smooth Endoplasmic Reticulum—collection of membranes that are smooth (no ribosomes). Helps make lipids. (Part of manufacturing plant of cell city)

Golgi Apparatus—collection of membranes that receive and modify products sent from the rough and smooth ER. The products are packaged into secretory vesicles which are shipped out. The golgi also produces lysosomes. (The golgi is the U.S. Postal Service of the cell city)

Lysosomes—round sacs of digestive enzymes. They can digest cell parts/materials or the cell itself. (The waste disposal service of the cell city)

Peroxisomes—round sac that contains enzymes for detoxification of drugs and alcohol. (Part of the waste disposal service of the cell city)

Mitochondria—rod or kidney bean shaped organelle that makes energy in the form of ATP. (Power plant of the cell city)

Other noteworthy organelles/structures:

Centrioles—help form mitotic spindle during cell division.

Flagellum—whip-like structure that allows the cell to move. (Sperm tails)

Cilia—long hair-like structures that move substances across the cell surface.

Microvilli—tiny hair-like structures that allow more surface area for absorption of nutrients.

The cell is like a city:

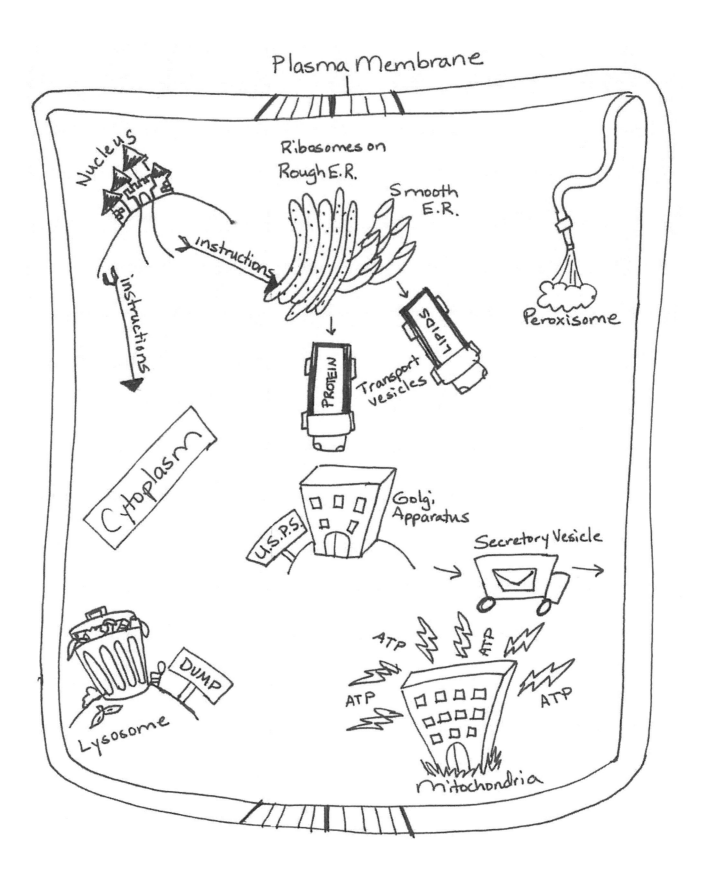

CHAPTER 2

Homeostasis and Feedback Loops

Homeostasis=Equilibrium or Balance.

Simple right? So we're done? Uhhh NO!

It truly is that simple, but we do need to delve a little deeper. Homeostasis is just about the most important concept to understand when studying physiology. Physiology can be defined as a set group of reactions that serve to maintain homeostasis. Homeostasis can be defined as the body's ability to remain stable internally under varying external conditions. As you are likely aware, your body doesn't match the temperature of your external environment. If it is 106 degrees Fahrenheit outside, does your body change to match that temperature? If it is 11 degrees Fahrenheit outside, does your body fluctuate to match that temperature?

NO! Of course not!

Imagine the havoc those changes would wreak on your organs? How could we expect our bodies to function in a normal capacity if the internal environment was changing with our surroundings? The body needs stability to function properly: temperature, pH, blood sugar, etc., all have checkpoints that the body must regulate. This does not mean, however, that the body can't fluctuate from the checkpoint that is homeostasis. There is a limited range of fluctuation that the body works within. The body uses two mechanisms to help maintain homeostatic regulation: negative feedback and positive feedback.

Negative Feedback

Negative feedback is a mechanism which strives to keep the variable in question (temperature, pH) close to the set checkpoint.

In plain English: Negative feedback resists change (or negative feedback feels negatively about change)!

The textbook example for this is thermoregulation. In other words, your body has a checkpoint for temperature, 98.6 degrees Fahrenheit. When you become overheated, receptors in the body notify the control center (the brain) which will activate the effector, or in this case, sweat glands. Vasodilation of blood vessels will occur. When sweat evaporates off the skin, heat is lost to the environment. In vasodilation, the blood vessels widen and therefore blood flows closer to the surface of the skin allowing heat to be lost into the surrounding air. A good analogy for this process is negative feedback in a thermostat.

Negative feedback in a thermostat:

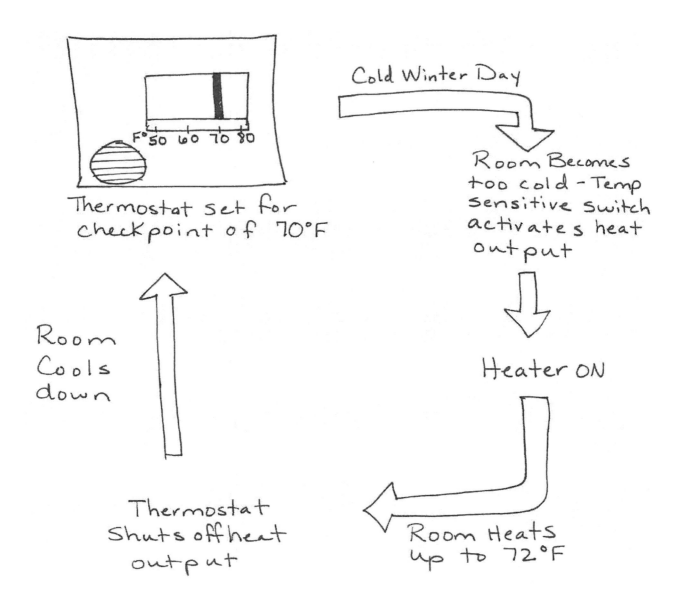

Thermostat set for checkpoint of 70°F

Cold Winter Day

Room Becomes too cold - Temp sensitive switch activates heat output

Heater ON

Room Heats up to 72°F

Thermostat Shuts off heat output

Room Cools down

Positive Feedback

Positive feedback exaggerates change. Meaning that we move further from checkpoint. Positive feedback can produce rapid change.

Wait! I thought we just said that we need to be close to checkpoint for our body to function properly. Now you are saying in positive feedback we are getting further away from checkpoint? Isn't this bad?

No! There are some instances in which this is necessary.

In plain English: Positive feedback amplifies change (or feels positively about change)!

Positive feedback in labor and delivery:

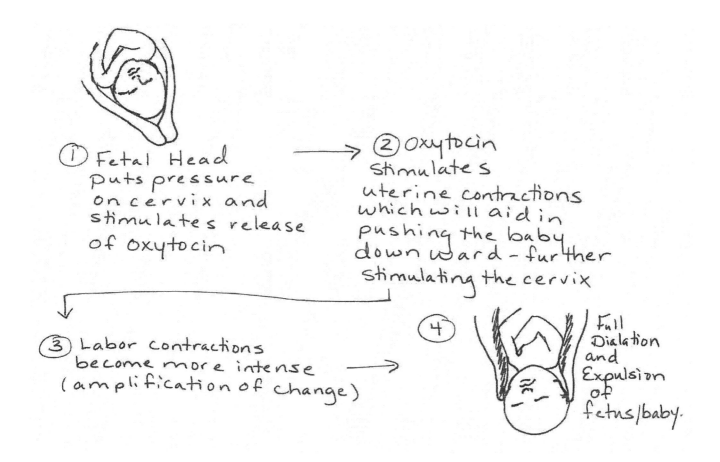

① Fetal Head puts pressure on cervix and stimulates release of Oxytocin → ② Oxytocin stimulates uterine contractions which will aid in pushing the baby downward - further stimulating the cervix

③ Labor contractions become more intense (amplification of change) →

④ Full Dialation and Expulsion of fetus/baby.

Transcription and Translation

If you recall from your general biology course, protein is a pretty big deal! Remember that the four biological molecules of life are protein, carbohydrate, nucleic acid, and lipids.

Protein accounts for so many important parts of our body: hair, skin, nails, muscle, bone, eye lens, enzymes, hormones, etc. Since all of those things are ridiculously important, we'd better be making new protein all the time! How do we do that? We do it by the process of transcription and translation! Say what?

Okay here's how it goes…

Transcription

Transcription is the process of copying the genetic instructions for how to make a protein from DNA to RNA.

FLASHBACK

DNA=Deoxyribonucleic Acid

RNA=Ribonucleic Acid

*Proteins are made of chains of amino acids

DNA Nitrogenous Bases	RNA Nitrogenous Bases
A=Adenine	A=Adenine
C=Cytosine	C=Cytosine
G=Guanine	G=Guanine
T-Thymine	U=Uracil
*A binds with T	*A binds with U
C binds with G	C binds with G

So why can't we just use DNA from the nucleus to make protein if that's where the instructions are? Why the extra step of creating RNA? DNA is too large to leave the nucleus (remember it's a double helix). RNA is a single strand that can fit through the tiny pores of the nuclear membrane and sneak out into the cytoplasm. RNA will carry out the instructions we need to make protein. Okay, so how does it start?

Transcription begins when a special enzyme called <u>RNA polymerase</u> (anything that ends in –ase is an enzyme) that binds to the DNA and transcribes (copies) it into a strand of RNA. It is a type of RNA called <u>mRNA </u>or messenger RNA. Imagine RNA polymerase as a typewriter.

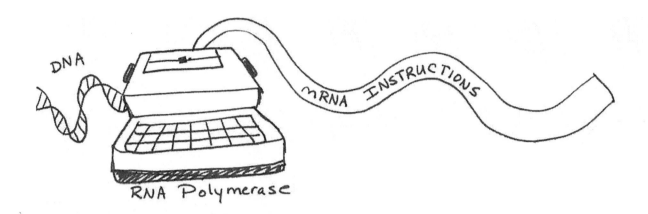

Once the mRNA is produced, it has to be modified and polished up to be ready to be translated. Once it is modified, it is ready to move into the cytoplasm with its genetic message for how to make protein.

<u>Translation</u>

Imagine that the mRNA, which is carrying genetic instructions for making protein, is in a foreign language and we need to translate it into English. This is the same idea used in translating the genetic instructions into amino acids or the subunits of protein (which by the way is what we are trying to make)! We're going to need some help here. Enter ribosomes!

The ribosome binds to the mRNA strand in the cytoplasm and begins translating the genetic code into protein when it reaches the <u>start codon</u>. The what? The start codon is the first three letters on the mRNA strand where protein begins to be made. The start codon is AUG. Remember what those letters stand for? (See flashback) Once the ribosome binds to the mRNA strand, <u>tRNA</u> enters the picture (tRNA=transfer RNA). Transfer RNA is in the business of transferring amino acids (hence the clever name). On one end, the tRNA carries an amino acid, and on the other is an anticodon or the complimentary group to the codon mentioned before.

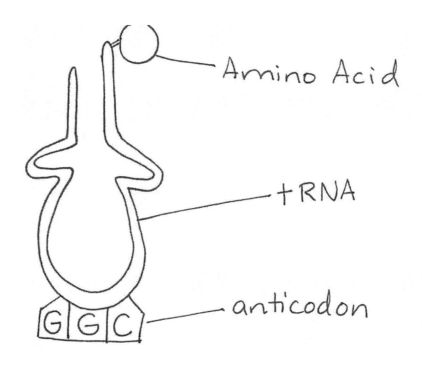

If the ribosome reads a codon CCG, it will look for a tRNA with the complimentary anticodon of GGC. It will bind this tRNA and then read the next codon, ex. AAC. The corresponding tRNA with complimentary anticodon UUG binds. Now the ribosome holds two tRNAs. The amino acids that each tRNA are carrying link together with a peptide bond, and the first bound tRNA releases. The mRNA continues to be read adding amino acids to a growing chain until the stop codon is reached to end the process (a stop codon like UGA). Once we've reached the stop codon the newly formed polypeptide/protein is released and the ribosome breaks apart. Mission accomplished!

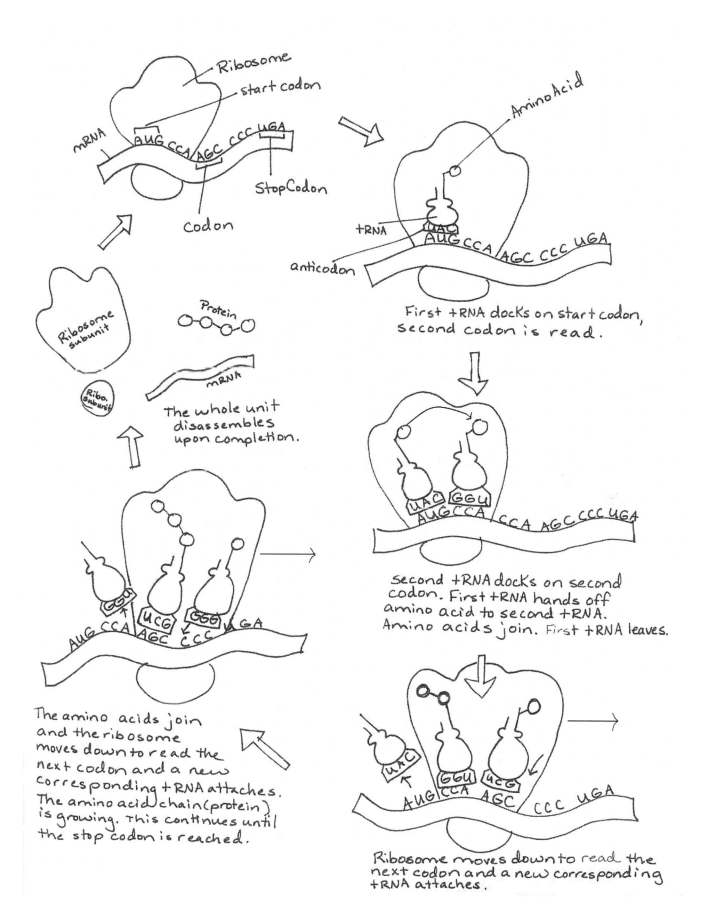

Ribosome
start codon
mRNA
AUG CCA AGC CCC UGA
StopCodon
codon

Amino Acid
tRNA
UAC
AUG CCA AGC CCC UGA
anticodon

First tRNA docks on start codon,
second codon is read.

Ribosome subunit
Protein
Ribo. Subunit
mRNA

The whole unit disassembles upon completion.

GGU
UAC GGU
AUG CCA CCA AGC CCC UGA

Second tRNA docks on second codon. First tRNA hands off amino acid to second tRNA. Amino acids join. First tRNA leaves.

GGU
UCG
GGU
AUG CCA AGC CCC UGA

The amino acids join and the ribosome moves down to read the next codon and a new corresponding tRNA attaches. The amino acid chain (protein) is growing. This continues until the stop codon is reached.

UAC
GGU UCG
AUG CCA AGC CCC UGA

Ribosome moves down to read the next codon and a new corresponding tRNA attaches.

CHAPTER 4

Tissue Review

Histology is the study of tissues. Tissues are collections of cells that work together to perform specific functions. There are 4 primary tissue types. Just remember, "Cats Eat Nervous Mice."

Connective

Epithelial

Nervous

Muscular

Let's examine the high points of each type.

Epithelial

- Covers and lines internal and external body surfaces (ex. inside of stomach AND outside of stomach).

- It is avascular (no blood vessels).

- Since it lines and covers, its main function is protection.

- It sits on a basement membrane that attaches it to underlying connective tissue.

- There are two main categories: simple and stratified.

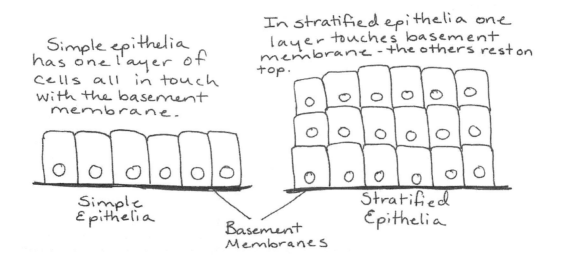

Simple epithelia has one layer of cells all in touch with the basement membrane.

In stratified epithelia one layer touches basement membrane - the others rest on top.

Simple Epithelia

Stratified Epithelia

Basement Membranes

There are three main shapes the cells can have: <u>squamous, cuboidal, columnar</u>.

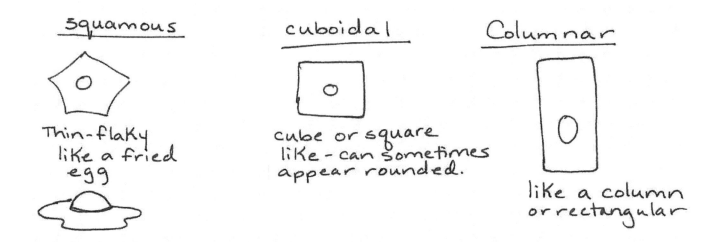

Connective

Connective tissue is called so because it connects organs to each other. Connective tissue is SOOOO different from epithelial. It has two main ingredients:

- Specialized cells

- Matrix (which is composed of <u>ground substance and fibers</u>)

The specialized cells will be different depending on what tissue we are examining. The matrix is what the cells are suspended in. This would be sort of like those bad jello salads…

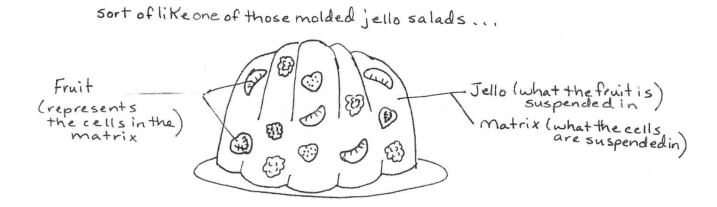

Unlike epithelia, which is almost entirely cells in direct contact with one another, connective tissue contains a lot of matrix with cells sprinkled about.

Connective tissue functions in:

- Support (bones and cartilage)

- Protection (bones and fat)

- Movement (bones and cartilage)

- Transport (blood)

- Storage (fat)

- Heat production (fat)

- Immune protection (immune cells)

Connective Tissue Types

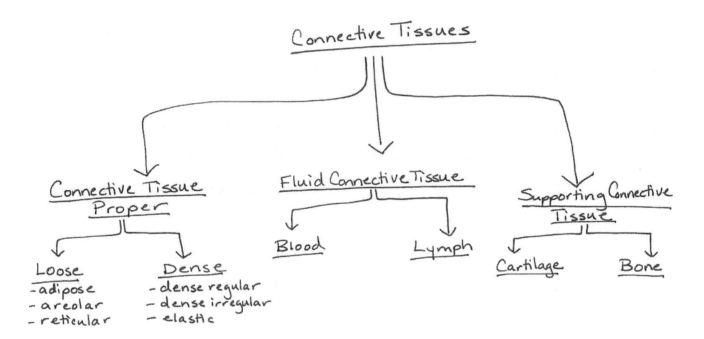

<u>Connective Tissue Proper High Points:</u>

- Has a varied cell population (lots of different types). Connective tissue proper types may have all or some of the cells mentioned below.

  <u>Fibroblasts-</u>keep the ground substance (part of the matrix that the cells are suspended in) syrupy.

  <u>Macrophages-</u>defenders of cells (think of them as tiny infection fighting soldiers).

  <u>Leukocytes-</u>also defenders of cells (they patrol for infection causing agents and toxins).

  <u>Plasma cells-</u>make antibodies to fight infection.

  <u>Mast cells-</u>found near blood vessels and secrete heparin for blood clotting and histamine for inflammation or increased blood flow.

  <u>Adipocytes-</u>fat cells.

- There are three types of fibers in connective tissue—helping to make up the matrix.

  <u>Collagen-</u>tough, stretchy and flexible.

  <u>Reticular-</u>sponge-like surrounding for organs.

  <u>Elastic-</u>extremely flexible and stretchy.

Defining the types of connective tissue proper:

<u>Areolar-</u> found in almost every part of the body. It surrounds blood vessels and is found as a packing material in small spaces of muscles, tendons and other tissues. It contains all six of the previously defined cells and all three fibers in its matrix.

<u>Reticular-</u>forms the structural framework of organs and is made largely of reticular fibers, fibroblasts and blood cells.

<u>Adipose-</u>fat tissue. Largely contains adipocytes.

<u>Dense regular connective tissue-</u>contains closely packed collagen fibers that are parallel. Found in tendon and ligaments.

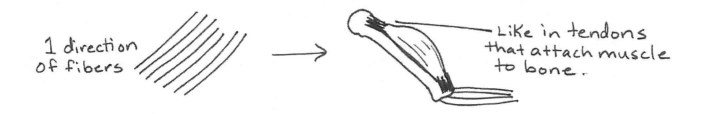

1 direction of fibers → Like in tendons that attach muscle to bone.

<u>Dense irregular connective tissue</u>-contains collagen that runs in random directions or irregular directions (hence the name). Found in the dermis of the skin.

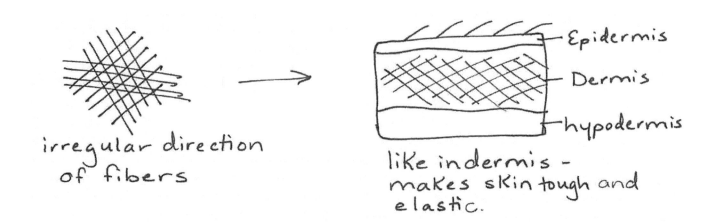

<u>Elastic tissue</u>-contains collagen and elastic fibers. Very stretchy and often found in places like the vocal cords.

<u>Fluid Connective Tissue High Points:</u>

There are two types of fluid connective tissue, blood and lymph. Each is watery and flows through tubular vessels.

<u>Blood-</u>works to transport oxygen and carbon dioxide throughout the body. It is composed of two things: formed elements (which is code for red blood cells, white blood cells and platelets) and plasma (which is the ground substance those cells are suspended in).

<u>Lymph-</u>lymph is formed when tissue fluids enter lymphatic vessels. It contains cells of the immune system that check for correct composition of lymph and respond to injury or infection.

<u>Supporting Connective Tissue High Points:</u>

Cartilage and bone are both supporting connective tissues. They support and give structure to the body. The matrix of both is typically very fibrous.

<u>Cartilage-</u>Cartilage has a firm gel matrix and contains lots of fibers and a fancy mineral called chondroitin sulfate. The primary cells are called <u>chondrocytes</u>. There are three types of cartilage:

Hyaline

Clear and contains fine collagen fibers that are widely spaced. Usually found in joint cavities.

Fibrocartilage

Densely packed collagen fibers, super tough. Makes up the intervertebral discs of vertebral column.

Elastic

Contains elastic fibers that form a tight mesh. Super flexible and tough. Found in external ear (go ahead, ball up your ear and let go—it will bounce back)!

Cool.

Bone-The matrix is made largely of collagen and calcium salts with bone cells interspersed. There are two types of bone: spongy and compact bone.

Spongy

Fills the tips of long bones, has a sponge like appearance and can withstand forces from all directions.

Compact

More dense and forms the external surfaces of all bones. Can withstand forces from limited direction.

Nervous Tissue

The nervous tissue is made of neurons (nerve cells) and protective cells called glial cells (we'll get to the details of this later in the nervous system review). The task of the nervous system is to direct and transmit stimuli.

Muscular Tissue

The muscular tissue is a contracting tissue that can direct movement of bones, digestive organs, urinary organs and blood in the vessels. There are three primary muscle types:

<u>Skeletal</u>	<u>Smooth</u>	<u>Cardiac</u>
Long spindle shaped cells	Short fat spindles	Branched
Multinucleate (more than one nucleus)	One nucleus	One nucleus
Voluntarily controlled	Involuntarily controlled	Involuntarily controlled
Striated or banded	Lacks striations	Striated or banded
Found attached to bone	Found lining hollow organs (stomach, intestines etc.)	Found in heart

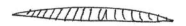 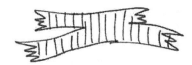

<u>Integumentary System</u>

The integumentary system includes the skin and accessory structures like hair, nails and glands. Its main functions are to protect the body from bacteria, viruses, UV light and other potential irritants. The skin is composed of two main layers. Under the two layers is a connective tissue layer. Just remember "Eat Delicious Honey."

E=epidermis

D=Dermis

H=Hypodermis

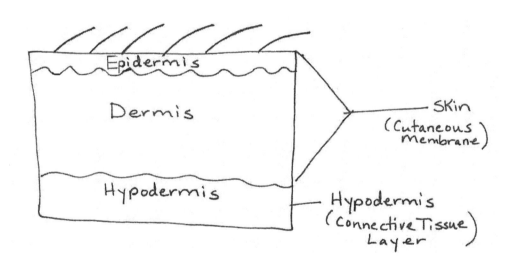

Skin can be classified as thick or thin based on the thickness of the epidermis. Thick skin would be found on the palms of the hands and soles of the feet. Thin skin would be found on all other parts of the body.

<u>Epidermis</u>

The epidermis is a stratified squamous epithelium (remember what that means)? The skin cells in the epidermis are called keratinocytes (anything that ends in –cyte is a cell). The cells are named so because they are filled with the protein keratin that serves to make the skin water resistant and tough. The epidermis is avascular (without blood vessels) because it is an epithelial tissue. It receives all nutrients and oxygen through the process of diffusion. This makes a ton of sense! Imagine if your epidermis were highly vascular, you could brush against a wall the wrong way and bleed like crazy! If the epidermis is meant to protect it, is best that it doesn't easily bleed. Avascular is the way to go here!

The epidermis itself can have four or five layers or zones called strata. There are four layers of strata in thin skin and five in thick skin. What does that mean? Check it out...

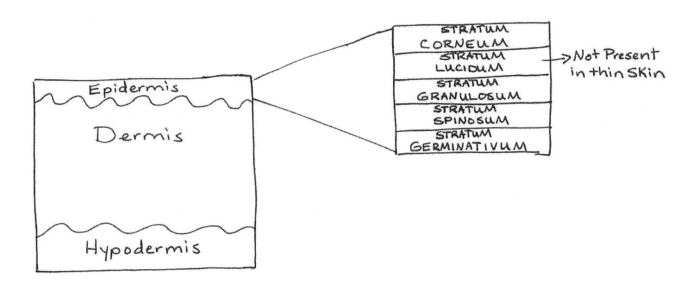

Stratum germinativum-made of one layer of cells that are constantly dividing to replace the cells that are flaking off from the top layer on a daily basis. We also find melanocytes (brown pigment producing cells that give the skin its color) and Merkel cells that are receptors for sensory information (feeling). Tip: just like plants germinate or reproduce, the germinativum is dividing or reproducing.

Stratum spinosum-is made of several layers of cells. At the top of this layer cells stop dividing, begin producing keratin, and flatten out.

Stratum granulosum-consists of three to five layers of flattened, densely packed keratinocytes.

Stratum lucidum-is a clear layer that is only seen in thick skin. Have you ever noticed the clear shiny nature of peeling calluses on the bottoms of your feet?

Stratum corneum-has up to 30 layers of dead, flaky and completely keratinized cells.

It takes one keratinocyte approximately one month to migrate from production in the stratum germinativum up to the stratum corneum to be shed. The keratinocyte will be slowly pushed up by the dividing layers underneath.

Dermis

The dermis is primarily made of collagen but also contains elastic and reticular fibers. Pinch your skin and pull it back! Did you see that bounce back? Remember to thank collagen, reticular, and elastic fibers! The dermis is highly vascular and also contains sweat, oil glands, hair and nails. The dermis has a raised and wavy surface that interlocks with the wavy bottom of the epidermis. They fit together like puzzle pieces to prevent sliding of the epidermis across the dermis. These ridges also cause fingerprints in the tips of the fingers.

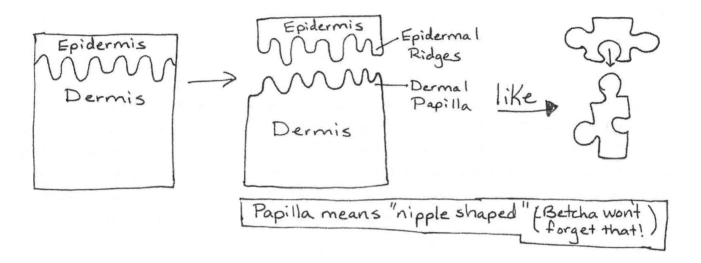

Hypodermis

The hypodermis (also called the subcutaneous layer) is made largely of adipose (fat) and areolar tissue. The hypodermis provides insulation for our bodies as well as padding and energy reserve in the form of fat. Hypodermic injections are given because the hypodermis is also highly vascular, which aids in quick absorption of drugs.

Skin color

Carotene is a yellow pigment found in yellow/orange vegetables like sweet potatoes and carrots. It gives the skin a yellow/orange hue based on the concentration in the skin.

Melanin is a brown/black pigment produced by melanocytes. The melanocytes are found in the stratum germinativum and spinosum. Melanocytes remind me of an octopus (check out the illustration). The amount of melanin produced by the skin is a combination of heredity and how much UV radiation you come in contact with. UV radiation is damaging to the skin and can cause mutations in the DNA of the keratinocytes. These mutations can lead to skin cancers that can be deadly. If you naturally have dark skin (not because of lying in a tanning bed mind you), then you are naturally better protected from UV radiation's mutating effects. How so?

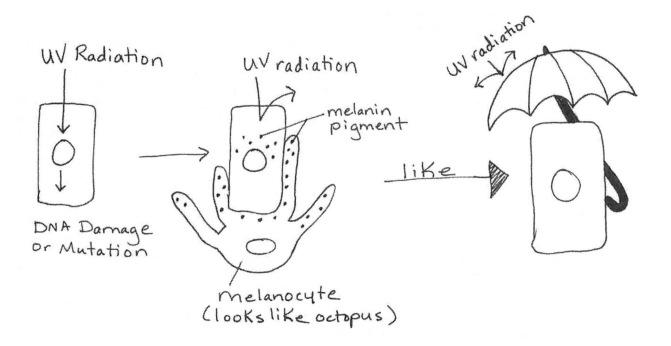

UV Radiation

DNA Damage
Or Mutation

UV radiation

melanin
pigment

melanocyte
(looks like octopus)

like

UV radiation

If you have to lie in the sun to become "tan," you are not naturally as well protected from UV radiation. The process of tanning is your body's way of telling you it is receiving UV radiation exposure. Even though some may think it looks pretty to have a tan, it can be damaging. Melanocytes are stimulated to produce melanin to protect the nucleus from mutation as seen above when they are exposed to UV radiation. The melanin pigments produced line up in front of the nucleus to shield it from the UV radiation that can damage the DNA in the nucleus. The collection of melanin pigments in the skin gives the skin a tan or brown color. Tans fade once the top layers of the pigmented stratum corneum shed off.

Hair

Hair is an accessory organ of the skin. Hair is composed mainly of dead keratinized cells.

There are two main types of hair: vellus and terminal. Vellus is the peach fuzz hair. It is soft and without color. It is found in places like the face in women and children. The terminal hair is coarse and has color. It is found in places like the eyebrows, scalp, facial hair and eyelashes. See the anatomy of a hair...

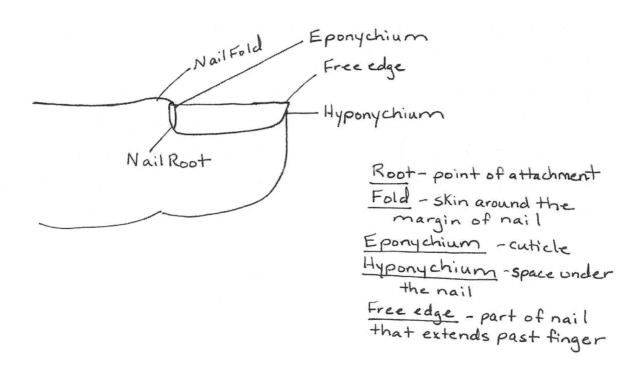

Follicle – tube shape – where hair grows
arrector pili – muscle stands hair on end
cuticle – jagged, dead coating
Shaft – hair above surface of skin
Root – hair within the follicle
Bulb – where hair originates
medulla – core
cortex – surrounds core

Labels on diagram: Shaft, cuticle, Sebaceous gland, Arrector Pili, Hair Follicle, Root, Hair Bulb, cortex, medulla, Hair Capillaries

Nails

Nails are also accessory organs of the integument. They are made of clear, thin, dead keratinized cells that are closely packed. See anatomy of a nail...

Labels on diagram: Nail Fold, Eponychium, Free edge, Hyponychium, Nail Root

Root – point of attachment
Fold – skin around the margin of nail
Eponychium – cuticle
Hyponychium – space under the nail
Free edge – part of nail that extends past finger

Glands

Sweat glands are also known as sudoriferous glands. There are two types: merocrine and apocrine. Merocrine glands release their products (sweat) by exocytosis (ejection out of the cell in a secretory vesicle). Apocrine glands release their products by a loss of cytoplasm with the secreted product.

Merocrine sweat is watery and odorless. Merocrine sweat glands are not associated with hair and open directly onto the skin surface. These sweat glands are found on most of the body. They are most concentrated on the soles of the feet, and palms of hands.

Apocrine sweat glands are typically associated with hair. These guys are called apocrine, but it has been found that they actually secrete in the style of merocrine glands. The glands discharge the sweat into a hair follicle. These glands are found in places like the armpit and groin. This sweat is more thick and contains fatty acids. Sweat that collects in areas like the arm pit becomes food for bacteria that then produces an unpleasant smell we call body odor. Bacterial gas??!! Ugh that's disgusting!

Sebaceous glands are oil glands. The fancy name for oil is sebum. They can open directly to the skin surface or they can open into a hair follicle like on the scalp. Oil glands are holocrine in nature. Holocrine means that the cells of the gland produce the product (oil), and then the cell breaks down spilling the product (oil) and various cell parts.

Ceruminous glands produce cerumen (ear wax). Ear wax coats the ear helping to make it water resistant and protects it from insects.

Mammary glands are milk glands. They typically only function under influence of lactation hormones. They are truly apocrine in nature.

Tissue Repair

1. Severed or broken blood vessels bleed and fill the cut. Helper cells like the mast cells move in and release histamine for inflammation. Inflammation brings in more blood and infection fighting antibodies.

2. Clotting begins to seal up the wound helping keep bacteria out. Macrophages begin to clean up the wound.

3. Granulation tissue forms. Granulation tissue is made of capillaries and fibroblasts which help to regenerate the connective tissue under the epidermis or epithelial tissue.

4. Cells of the stratum germinativum divide and migrate around the perimeter of the cut continuously dividing and healing from the inside out. Presto! The scab pops off.

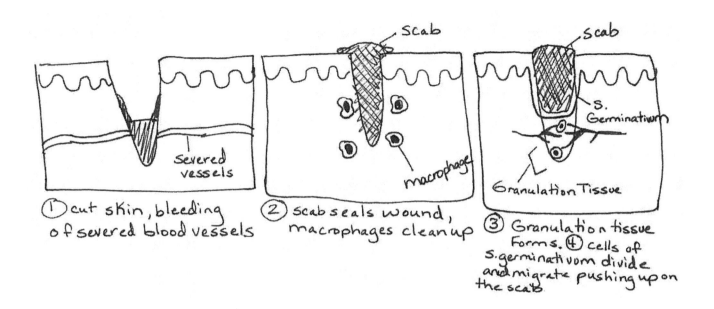

① cut skin, bleeding of severed blood vessels

② scab seals wound, macrophages clean up

③ Granulation tissue forms. ④ cells of S. germinativum divide and migrate pushing up on the scab.

CHAPTER 6

Osseous Tissue

<u>Osseous tissue</u> or bone is a supporting connective tissue that has a dense mineralized matrix. Bone aids the body in support, stability and protection. Before we delve into the specifics of the tissue itself, let's look at bone shapes: Life Is Forever Sacred.

L=Long

I=Irregular

F=Flat

S=Short

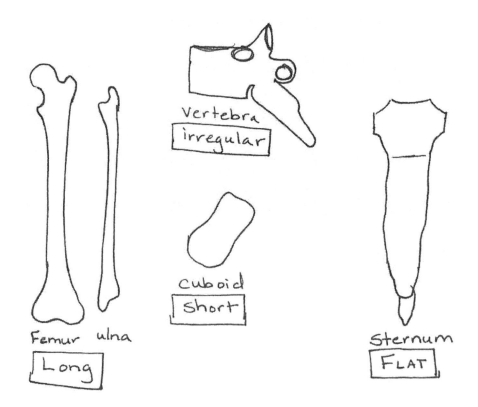

The main features of a long bone:

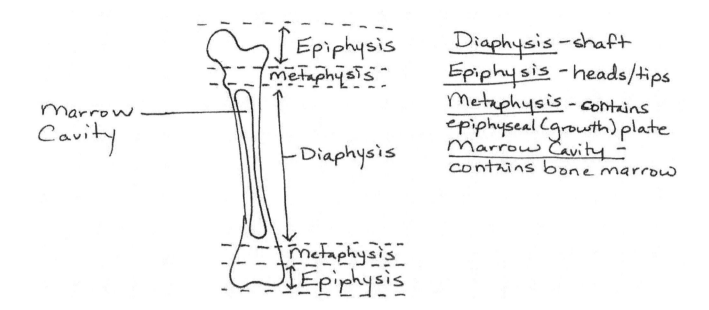

Diaphysis – shaft
Epiphysis – heads/tips
Metaphysis – contains epiphyseal (growth) plate
Marrow Cavity – contains bone marrow

There are two types of bone: compact or dense bone and spongy or cancellous bone. Dense bone is solid and spongy bone is how it sounds — kind of spongy! It's not squishy like a kitchen sponge but it has the appearance of a kitchen sponge. The bone is loosely arranged and porous. Each type of bone serves a very important purpose. Compact bone can handle stress best in one or limited directions (like your weight). Compact bone typically covers bones and has a solid appearance. Spongy can handle stress from multiple directions by absorbing impact. Spongy bone is typically found at the ends of long bones and in the middle of most other bones. Spongy bone also helps to make our bones lighter. Together, compact and spongy bone make a tough skeleton.

Epiphyseal cartilage or the growth plate is located in the metaphysis region of the bones. It is made of cartilage and allows for growth in adolescence when stimulated by growth hormone. In adults the epiphyseal cartilage has sealed creating the epiphyseal line. Growth can no longer occur. In an X-Ray, bone shows up but cartilage appears black.

Here is a child's X-Ray in comparison to an adults X-Ray.

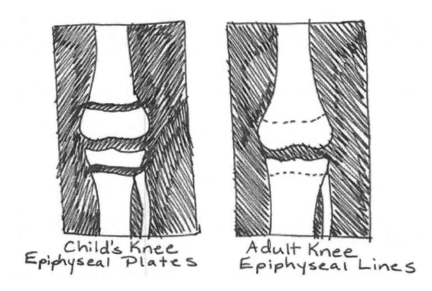

Child's Knee
Epiphyseal Plates

Adult Knee
Epiphyseal Lines

Now let's get into the makeup of the osseous tissue. Recall that bone or osseous tissue is a supporting connective tissue. Also remember that all connective tissue is made of specialized cells and a matrix (ground substance and fibers) that those cells are suspended in. The specialized cells:

Osteoprogenitor cells-differentiate into osteoblasts and are important in the repair of fractures.

Osteoblasts-make or "blast" out new bone matrix.

Osteocytes-"mature" bone cells. These guys were osteoblasts but have trapped themselves in the matrix they have created. They maintain the protein and mineral content of the matrix.

Osteoclasts-are cells that dissolve bone.

The matrix of bone is made largely of calcium and collagen fibers. More specifically bone is made from hydroxyapatite (calcium salt), sodium, magnesium and fluoride. The calcium salt portion of bone is very hard but extremely brittle; whereas, the collagen portion of bone is strong and flexible but cannot stand up to compression. Together the calcium portion and the collagen portion make a tough resilient tissue.

We will now examine the differences between spongy bone and compact bone. The functional unit of compact bone is the osteon. In an osteon, the osteocytes are arranged in layers of matrix (lamellae) around a central canal. The central canal contains one or more blood vessels that nourish the osteon. The osteocytes each live in pockets sandwiched in the matrix called lacunae. Think of the lacunae as the osteocytes' little house. Just like in a neighborhood or subdivision, the houses are connected by streets. The "streets" of the osteon are the canaliculi. Canaliculi are narrow "streets" that pass through the matrix and attach the lacunae to each other and the nearby blood vessels. This arrangement aids in the sharing of nutrients and gases. The canaliculi contain cytoplasmic extensions (sort of like tentacles) of the osteocytes so that the osteocytes can communicate and share with one another.

Osteon as a neighborhood:

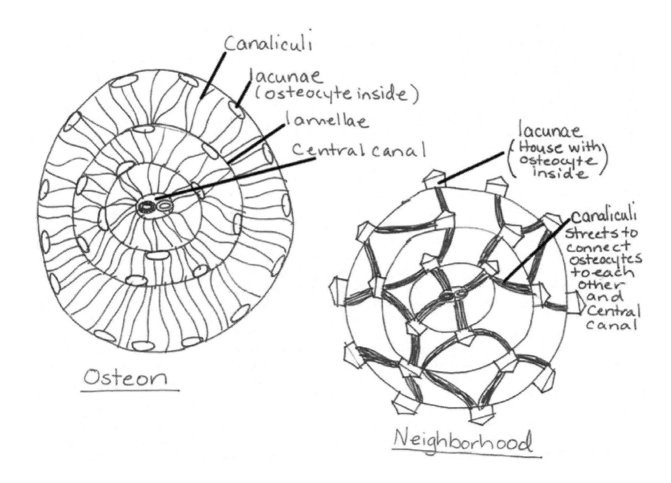

Osteon

Neighborhood

In spongy bone the lamellae are not arranged in osteons. The matrix of spongy bone is strut-like and forms a sponge-like pattern called <u>trabeculae</u>. Spongy bone is avascular and must receive nutrients and gases by diffusion. <u>Red bone marrow</u> is found in spongy bone. Red bone marrow is responsible for blood cell formation. Spongy bone may also contain <u>yellow bone marrow</u> which is largely fat and provides an energy source.

A <u>periosteum</u> is a membrane that covers compact bone. It is made of fibers and an inner layer of osteoprogenitor cells. It separates the bone from other tissues and helps with bone growth and repair. The <u>endosteum</u> is a layer of osteoprogenitor cells that line the marrow cavity and help with bone growth and repair. In areas where there are no osteoprogenitor cells in the marrow cavity, you will find osteoclasts and osteoblasts remodeling the matrix.

Ossification

Ossification is the formation of bone. There are two types of ossification to cover: intramembranous and endochondral.

Intramembranous ossification will generate the flat bones of the skull and the majority of the clavicle or collar bone. We begin with embryonic mesenchymal tissue (fetal tissue). Cells of the embryonic tissue begin to differentiate into osteoblasts that will produce the matrix of the developing bone. The developing bone grows outward in little projections called spicules. Blood vessels begin to be trapped by the forming bone spicules. At first the bone formed is largely spongy bone. Continuous remodeling will produce osteons that are the units of compact bone. Endochondral ossification starts with tiny cartilage (hyaline) models of the bones to be. These cartilage models will be converted to bone in the process of endochondral ossification. The cartilage models enlarge and the matrix of the cartilage will begin to calcify. Blood vessels grow into the shaft of the cartilage model. The cells in this region differentiate into osteoblasts and cover the shaft of the cartilage model in a thin layer of bone. The blood supply migrates further into the shaft of the cartilage model and more osteoblasts differentiate. The new osteoblasts begin to produce spongy bone in the shaft of the cartilage model. This is called the primary ossification center. This bone development will spread towards the ends of the cartilage model. The shaft of the model is now filled with spongy bone. The bone enlarges, osteoclasts dissolve away some of the spongy bone to form a marrow cavity. Next, the center of the epiphyses begins to calcify and more blood vessels move into the area. These areas are called the secondary ossification centers. The epiphyses will be filled with spongy bone except for the surface of the bone, which will remain cartilage to pad the joint cavity. The epiphyseal cartilage will also remain so that the bones may continue to grow after birth.

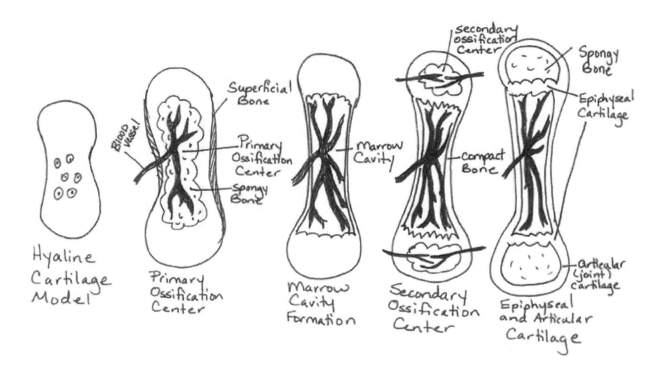

<u>Blood Calcium</u>

Bones continue to grow and remodel throughout life. Vitamin D is converted to <u>calcitriol</u>. Calcitriol behaves as a hormone and helps the small intestine absorb phosphate and calcium and limits the excretion of calcium and phosphate through urination. Calcitriol can also activate osteoclasts.

<u>Calcitonin</u> and <u>parathyroid hormone (PTH)</u> both play a role in blood calcium levels. When your blood calcium is TOO HIGH, calcitonin will lower it. Remember: Calcitonin TONES DOWN blood calcium. Calcitonin causes the osteoclasts to limit their activity (less bone dissolving). This means less calcium is being taken from the skeleton and added to blood. Calcitonin helps the kidneys to allow calcium loss through urination. These two actions combined with less absorption of calcium in the kidney due to lowered PTH will cause the blood calcium levels to decline.

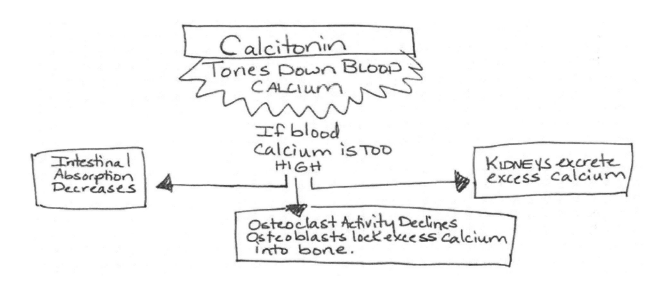

Parathyroid hormone or PTH helps raise blood calcium when it is TOO LOW. PTH causes osteoclasts to become active and remove calcium from the skeleton to incorporate into the blood. PTH also enhances the action of calcitriol so that the rate of intestinal absorption increases. Finally, PTH decreases the rate of kidney excretion of calcium.

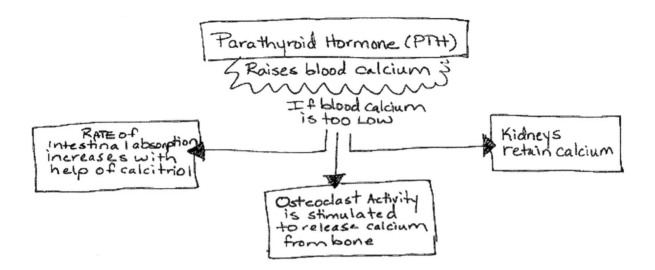

Healing Bone

Right after the fracture occurs, the bone begins to bleed. A large blood clot (fracture hematoma) forms. The fracture causes the endosteum and periosteum to undergo cell division. The newly produced cells migrate to the fracture and an external callus (cartilage and bone) forms and surrounds the fracture. The cartilage at the center of the external callus begins to convert to spongy bone. An internal callus of spongy bone begins to form within the marrow cavity. At that point, the fracture is well braced for continued healing. Broken and dead bits of bone are removed. Spongy bone begins to unite the broken ends along the fracture line. The surrounding area will be remodeled as the bone of the callus begins to diminish, being replaced with compact bone.

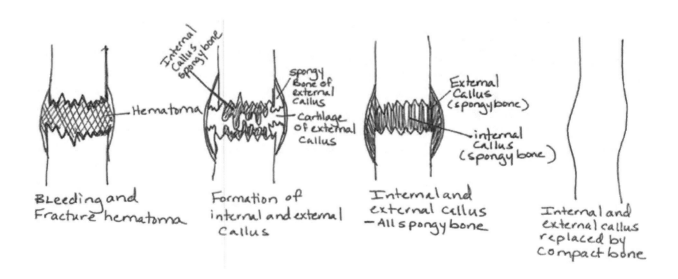

Fracture types

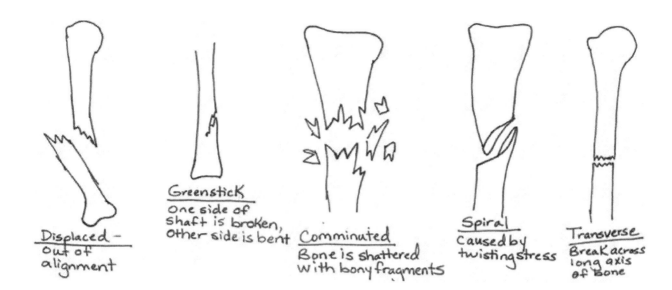

Displaced –
Out of
alignment

Greenstick
One side of
Shaft is broken,
Other side is bent

Comminuted
Bone is shattered
with bony fragments

Spiral
Caused by
twisting stress

Transverse
Break across
long axis
of Bone

Osteopenia and Osteoporosis

Osteopenia is defined as inadequate ossification. This happens to all of us as we age naturally. As we age, our osteoblast activity slows down. The problem here is that our osteoclast activity stays the same which means that we begin to lose bone mass over time. When the bone mass declines enough to affect normal function, we call this osteoporosis. Bone affected by osteoporosis is very fragile and likely to break under minimal stress.

CHAPTER 7

Axial Skeleton

A Flythrough to Complement Your Lab Study

NOTE: This chapter is to be read alongside your lab atlas/manual so that you may examine the bones and structures for the lab portion of your course.

The axial skeleton makes up the center axis of the body. It is what your appendages (arms and legs) attach to. The axial skeleton is made up of: Apples Have Very Tasty Skin.

A=Auditory Ossicles (Bones of ear)

H=Hyoid bone

V=Vertebral Column

T=Thoracic (rib) cage

S=Skull

The axial skeleton gives the body structural support and protects vital organs like the spinal cord, brain, lungs and heart. The axial skeleton also provides surfaces for muscle attachment.

Skull

The skull contains 22 bones and functions in protection of the brain. Almost all skull bones are attached by sutures. A suture is an immoveable connection between the skull bones where the bones are joined by tough connective tissue.

As you begin studying for your axial skeleton lab you will notice the terms foramen or foramina and fissures. Foramen or foramina and fissures are passageways for nerves and blood vessels.

Auditory Ossicles and Hyoid Bone

The auditory ossicles or bones of the ear will be further discussed in the special senses review. The hyoid bone helps support the larynx, pharynx and tongue.

Vertebral Column

The vertebral column is made of 26 bones. There are 24 vertebrae, 1 sacrum and 1 coccyx. There are 5 vertebral regions: cervical, thoracic, lumbar, sacral and coccygeal.

Cervical vertebrae=7 (Cervical vertebra 1 is called the atlas and cervical vertebra 2 is called the axis)

Thoracic vertebrae=12

Lumbar vertebrae=5

During development, the sacrum begins as a group of 5 vertebrae and the coccyx begins with 3-5 small vertebrae. Usually the vertebrae of the sacrum fuse by age 25-30 and the ossification of the coccyx varies.

Thoracic Cage

The thoracic cage consists of the thoracic vertebrae, ribs, and sternum or breastbone. There are 12 pairs of ribs.

CHAPTER 8

Appendicular Skeleton

A Flythrough to Complement Your Lab Study

NOTE: This chapter is to be read alongside your lab atlas/manual so that you may examine the bones and structures for the lab portion of your course.

The appendicular skeleton includes the limbs and the girdles. The limbs, as in the bones of the legs and arms and the girdles, as in what attaches those legs and arms to the axial skeleton. The appendicular skeleton has two girdles: The pectoral girdle and the pelvic girdle.

Pectoral Girdle

Each arm joins to the axial skeleton at the pectoral or shoulder girdle. The pectoral girdle is made up of the scapula or shoulder blade and the clavicle or collar bone. The bones of the arm include the humerus, ulna, radius, carpals, metacarpals, and phalanges. The humerus is the upper arm bone and the ulna and radius make up the forearm. The radius lines up with the thumb and the ulna lines up with the pinky finger. Remember T. Rex and P. U.!

T=Thumb

R=Radius

P=Pinky

U=Ulna

To remember the bones of the wrist or carpals remember: She Likes Topping Pizza (with) Tasty Tomatoes Cheese and Ham.

S=Scaphoid

L=Lunate

T=Triquetrum

P=Pisiform

T=Trapezium

T=Trapezoid

C=Capitate

H=Hamate

The metacarpals attach to the carpals and are named with Roman numerals I-V. Roman numeral I is the thumb and Roman numeral V is the pinky finger. The thumb or pollex has two phalange bones and the rest of the fingers each have three.

<u>Pelvic Girdle</u>

The bones of the pelvic girdle are much larger than those of the pectoral girdle. They must withstand the stress of weight bearing and our body movement. The pelvic girdle consists of the two hip bones. Keep in mind that the pelvic girdle is not the same as the pelvis.

The pelvic girdle consists of the two coxal bones or hip bones. Each hip bone is formed by the fusion of three bones: ilium, ischium and pubis. The two hip bones or coxal bones are joined by a pad of fibrocartilage called the pubic symphysis. (See your lab atlas/manual)

The <u>pelvis</u> consists of the two coxal bones AND the sacrum and coccyx. (See lab atlas/manual)

The lower limbs consist of the femur, tibia, fibula, patella, tarsals, metatarsals, and phalanges. The ankle or tarsus consists of seven tarsal bones. Just remember: <u>T</u>ess <u>C</u>aught <u>C</u>arl <u>L</u>ying <u>I</u>n <u>M</u>any <u>N</u>egotiations.

<u>T</u>alus

<u>C</u>alcaneus

<u>C</u>uboid

<u>L</u>ateral Cuneiform

<u>I</u>ntermediate Cuneiform

<u>M</u>edial Cuneiform

<u>N</u>avicular

The metatarsal bones are 5 bones that are, like the hand, numbered by Roman numerals I-V. Roman numeral I is the big toe or hallux and Roman numeral V is the pinky toe.

CHAPTER 9

<u>Articulations</u>

After covering the skeleton we must now understand how the skeleton is able to move. Muscle will play a role in this, however, joints or articulations are our current topic of discussion. A joint or <u>artic-ulation</u> is where two bones meet. Typically when we think of joints we think of movement. All joints do not move! Notice that movement is not part of the definition of joint or articulation. Articulations like the shoulder or elbow are moveable and weight bearing, whereas articulations like the sutures of the skull are immoveable and most useful for protection of organs and tissues. Articulations are classified by their movement:

<u>Articulations</u>

<u>Synarthrosis</u>

*Performs little or no movement

<u>Amphiarthrosis</u>

*Slightly moveable

<u>Diarthrosis</u>

*Freely moveable

Synarthroses, amphiarthroses and diarthroses can be held together by <u>fibrous</u>, <u>cartilaginous</u>, or <u>bony fusion</u> connections. In a fibrous connection collagen from the matrix of one bone grows into the matrix of another. In cartilaginous connections the two bones are bound by cartilage. In bony fusion connections the two bones were once separate and have now fused together with bone.

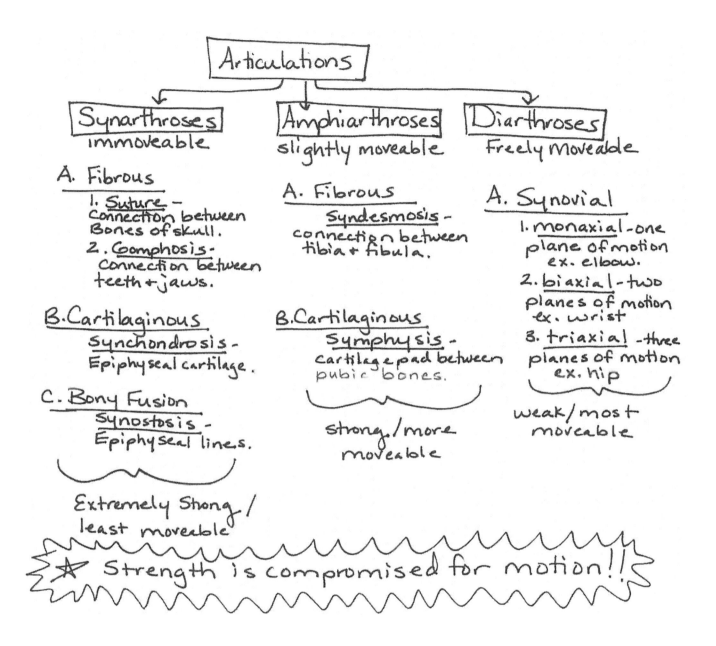

Articulations

Synarthroses
immoveable

A. Fibrous
1. Suture -
Connection between
Bones of skull.
2. Gomphosis-
Connection between
teeth + jaws.

B. Cartilaginous
Synchondrosis -
Epiphyseal cartilage.

C. Bony Fusion
Synostosis -
Epiphyseal lines.

Extremely Strong /
least moveable

Amphiarthroses
slightly moveable

A. Fibrous
Syndesmosis -
connection between
tibia + fibula.

B. Cartilaginous
Symphysis -
cartilage pad between
pubic bones.

strong. / more
moveable

Diarthroses
Freely Moveable

A. Synovial
1. monaxial - one
plane of motion
ex. elbow.
2. biaxial - two
planes of motion
ex. wrist
3. triaxial - three
planes of motion
ex. hip

weak / most
moveable

★ Strength is compromised for motion!!

The diarthroses or synovial joints allow for a much greater range of motion. Synovial joints are enclosed within a capsule called the <u>articular capsule</u> which is lined with a special membrane called the <u>synovial membrane</u>. The synovial membrane secretes <u>synovial fluid</u> to lubricate the joint. This is what we call joint fluid. In a synovial joint the ends of the bones or epiphyses are covered by a thin cartilage called <u>articular cartilage</u>. This cartilage soaks up synovial fluid. When the bones press together synovial fluid leaks out between them. The lubrication will allow the bones to slide past each other, greatly reducing friction. If the cartilage is damaged, friction will increase, causing severe pain.

An accessory structure found in the synovial joint is the <u>meniscus</u>. Menisci are pads of cartilage between opposing bones that act as little cushions. <u>Fat pads</u> are typically found on the outside of the articular capsule and act as insulation to the joint. <u>Ligaments</u> are very strong, connect the bones and strengthen the joints. <u>Bursae</u> are fluid filled pouches that form where a tendon or ligament rub against other tissues. Bursae can act as shock absorbers for the joint.

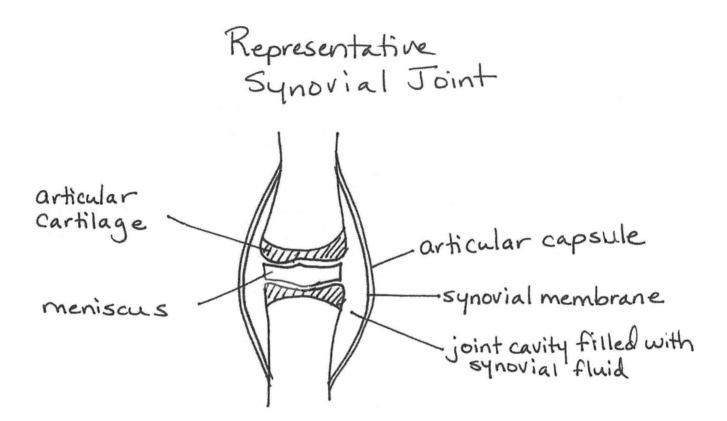

Dynamic Motion

<u>Linear motion/gliding</u> is when two surfaces slide past one another. This type of movement happens between bones of the carpals and tarsals.

<u>Angular motion</u> includes <u>extension</u>, <u>flexion</u>, <u>adduction</u>, <u>abduction</u> and <u>circumduction</u>. Flexion is when the movement reduces the angle between the articulating bones. Extension increases the angle between the articulating bones. When we stand in the anatomical position all of our major joints except the ankle are in extension. <u>Hyperextension</u> is when we extend past the anatomical position. Abduction is movement away from the body in the frontal plane. Moving it back to the anatomical position is adduction. (When a person is ABDUCT-ed they are taken AWAY, when something is ADDucted it is ADDED back). Circumduction is demonstrated when you move your arm in a circle. (Like drawing an invisible circle in the air with your arm).

Angular Motion

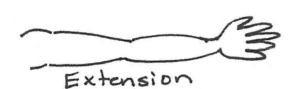

Extension

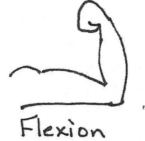

Flexion

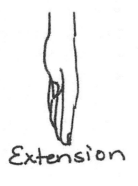

Extension

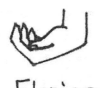

Flexion

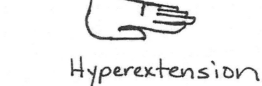

Hyperextension

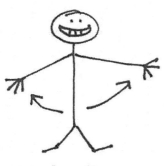

Abduction

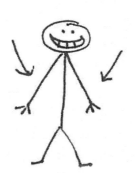

Adduction

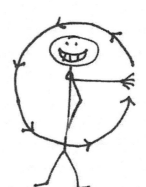

Circumduction

Rotation may include left or right rotation or pronation and supination.

Rotation

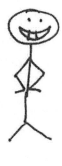 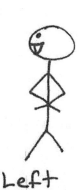 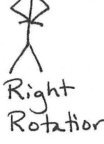 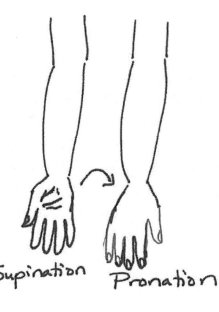

Left Rotation

Right Rotation

Supination   Pronation

Inversion is a motion of the foot that turns the foot inwards. Eversion is the opposite movement. Dorsiflexion is flexion of the ankle and points the toes upwards. Plantar flexion elevates the heel and points the toe downward (like a ballet toe).

Opposition is the movement of the thumb towards the tips of the other fingers. This movement is what allows us to hold objects.

Protraction is when you move a part of your body anteriorly. You protract your jaw when you give yourself an under bite. Retraction is the opposite of retraction or when you pull your jaw back in. Elevation is when you move a part superiorly; depression is when you move a part inferiorly.

Special Movements

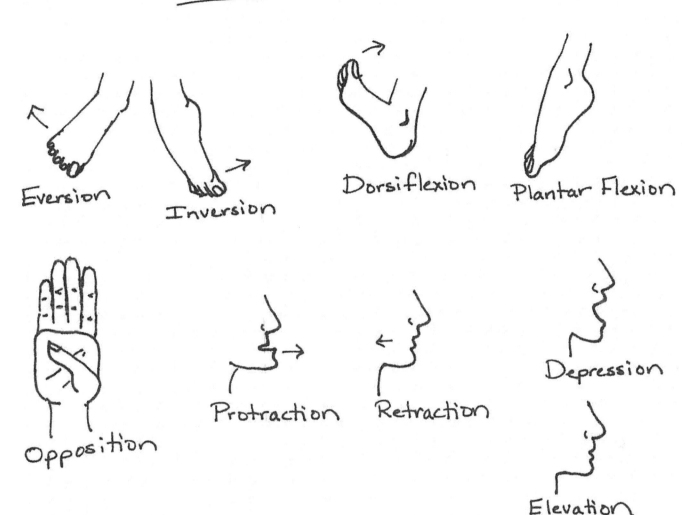

Types of Synovial Joints

Gliding joints usually involve flat articular surfaces that slide across each other. (ex. Carpals and tarsals)

Hinge joints allow motion in a single plane (monaxial) sort of like the hinge of a door. (ex. Elbow)

Pivot joints are monaxial and can only rotate. (ex. Atlas and axis)

Ellipsoidal joints form when one articular surface sits in another bone's concave articular surface. (ex. Radiocarpal joint)

Saddle joints fit together like a person sits on a saddle. (ex. First carpo-metacarpal joint)

Ball-and-socket joints have an articular surface with a rounded ball-like head that fits into a concave socket-like articular surface. (ex. Shoulder or hip)

Note: Please see your lab atlas/manual or textbook for anatomical structures of specific joints.

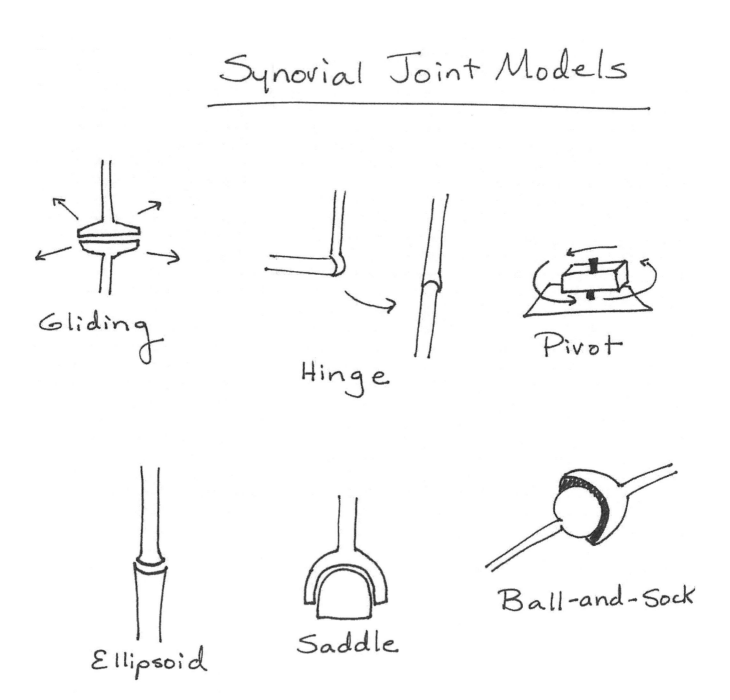

Synovial Joint Models

Gliding

Hinge

Pivot

Ellipsoid

Saddle

Ball-and-Sock

Joint Problems

As we age joint problems become more common. <u>Rheumatism</u> describes pain and stiffness of the muscular system and/or the skeleton. <u>Arthritis</u> is a condition involving wear and tear of the articular cartilage. <u>Osteoarthritis</u> specifically involves degeneration of the articular cartilage caused by advancing age or problems with collagen formation. <u>Rheumatoid arthritis</u> is an autoimmune condition where the joints become inflamed. Allergies, infection or genetics can be blamed for rheumatoid arthritis.

Muscle Characters.
- Excitable
- Contractile.
- Extensible
- Elastic

<u>Muscle Tissue</u>

of the four primary types of tissue. Muscle tissue is made of mainly traction. Remember that there are three types of muscle we previ- and smooth muscle. We will concentrate on skeletal muscle tissue

roduce movement by pulling on the bones of the skeleton—hence ft tissues, maintains our body position, guards entrances and exits ody temperature and stores nutrients.

Skeletal muscle is incredibly organized. The entire muscle (like the bicep) is surrounded by an <u>epimysium</u>. The epimysium is a layer of collagen that separates the muscle from other tissues. The <u>perimysium</u> divides the muscle into sections that contain <u>fascicles</u> which are bundles of muscle cells/fibers. Fascicles are separated from each other within a muscle by the perimysium. Muscle fascicles are the "grains" you see when you eat meat. Yum! The muscle fascicles are made of bundles of muscle cells/fibers. Those muscle cells/fibers are surrounded by an <u>endomysium</u>. The endomysium is made largely of areolar tissue and allows room for capillaries and nerves to reach each muscle fiber. These nerves will control the muscle. The collagen that is interwoven through the muscle converges to form a tendon that attaches to bone. If the muscle contracts it will pull on tendon that is attached to the bone and we have movement! Skeletal muscles can only contract if they are told to by the central nervous system or CNS.

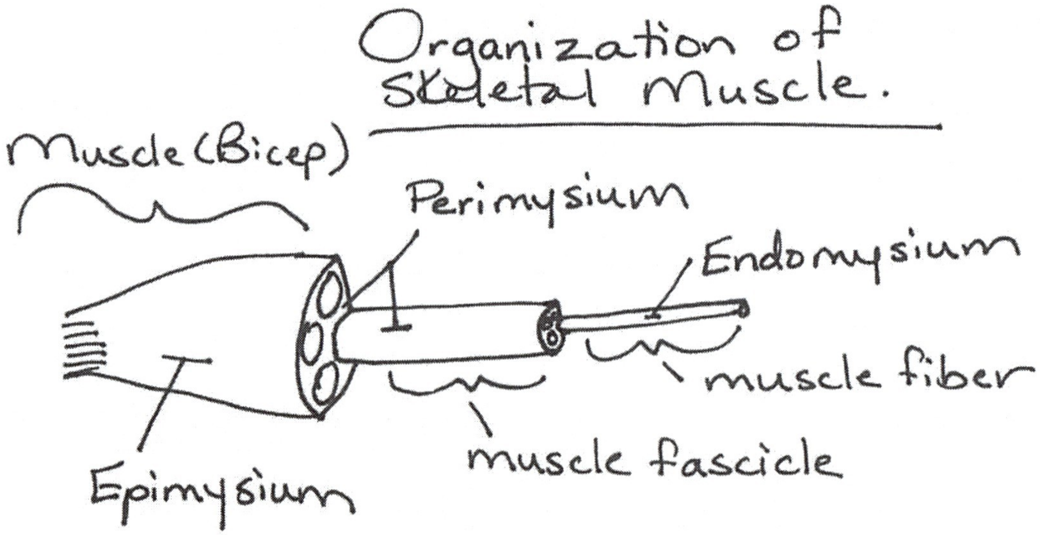

Organization of
Skeletal Muscle.

Muscle (Bicep)

Perimysium

Endomysium

muscle fiber

muscle fascicle

Epimysium

Skeletal Muscle Fiber Characteristics

Skeletal muscle fibers are super interesting because they have to be equipped for movement. This means that they will look quite a bit different from many other cells. In the cell world, muscle cells are giants! Some can even be seen with the naked eye! That's huge! Recall from the tissue chapter that they are also multinucleate (each cell can contain hundreds of nuclei), striated (striped appearance), and voluntary (we can control most of them).

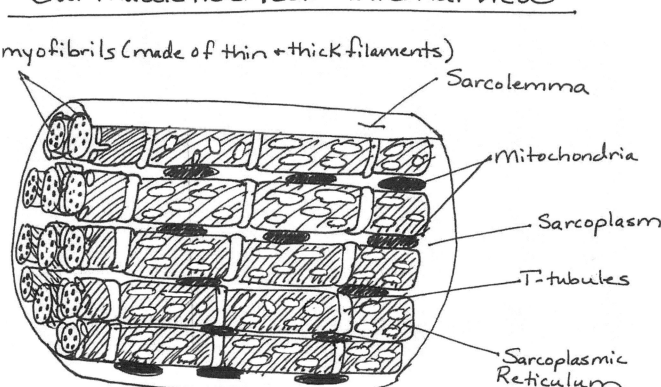

Cut muscle fiber/cell - internal view

myofibrils (made of thin + thick filaments)

Sarcolemma

Mitochondria

Sarcoplasm

T-tubules

Sarcoplasmic Reticulum

The skeletal muscle cell has a plasma membrane called the sarcolemma. The cell is filled with sarcoplasm or cytoplasm, and transverse tubules or T-tubules. The T-tubules are used to transmit signals (we'll discuss the purpose of this later). The T-tubules surround myofibrils which are as long as the cell. Myofibrils are made of two kinds of protein filaments, thin and thick filaments. Thin filaments are also known as actin and thick filaments are also known as myosin. If myofibrils are able to shorten, this will shorten the entire muscle—which is a contraction! Skeletal muscles are also chock full of mitochondria to make ATP that will power the contractions. The sarcoplasmic reticulum is a series of membranes that surrounds the myofibrils. The sarcoplasmic reticula store calcium ($Ca2+$) which will be used in contraction.

<u>Sarcomeres</u>

The tiny units of a myofibril are sarcomeres. They lie end to end on the myofibril. Sarcomeres are made up of the aforementioned thin and thick filaments or actin and myosin. When the actin and myosin interact, the sarcomeres will shorten, in turn shortening the myofibrils, and eventually the entire muscle. The sarcomeres are what give the muscle a striated or banded appearance. The thick filaments are located at the center of the sarcomere and are shown in the figure as thick black horizontal lines. The thin filaments are the thin horizontal lines on either side of the thick filaments in the figure. The area that contains the thick filaments entirely with a slight overlap of the thin filaments is called the <u>A band</u>. The thick filaments are held together by the <u>M line</u>. The <u>H band</u> surrounds the M line and contains only thick filaments. The <u>I band</u> contains only thin filaments and reaches from the A band of one sarcomere to the A band of the adjacent sarcomere. The <u>zone of overlap</u> is, like it sounds, the area where the thin and thick filaments overlap. The <u>Z line</u> marks the boundary between neighboring sarcomeres (it also looks like a zig zag which is how I remember 'Z'). <u>Titin</u> is an elastic protein that helps keep the thin and thick filaments lined up as well as helping with contraction and relaxation of the muscle.

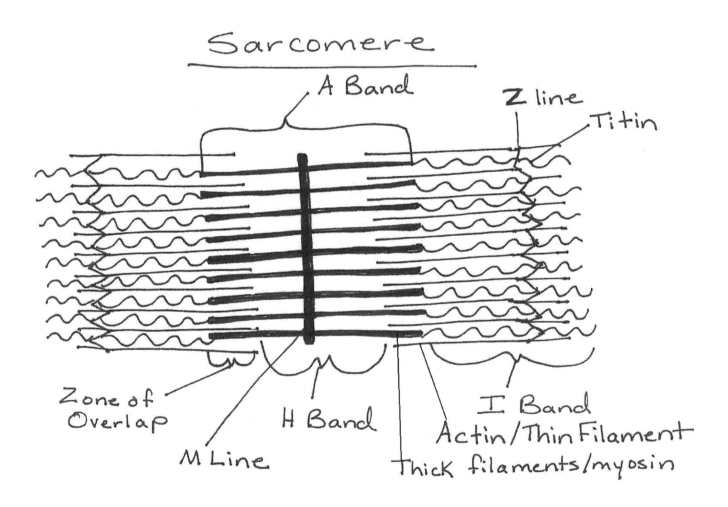

Thin Filament

Thin filaments or actin, contain 4 different proteins. The proteins are F-actin, nebulin, tropomyosin, and troponin. F-actin is a twisted strand of two rows of G-actin (it reminds me of two strands of pearls twisted together). Each G-actin molecule has an active or binding site on it that will become important later in the discussion of muscle contraction. Tropomyosin covers the actives sites on the G-actin molecules to prevent binding. Troponin is bound to tropomyosin.

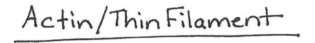

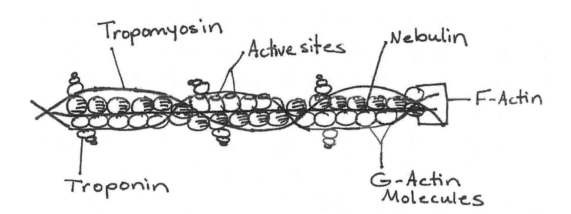

Thick Filaments

Thick filaments are made of twisted myosin subunits. The thick filaments are covered with myosin heads. The heads project outwards towards the thin filaments.

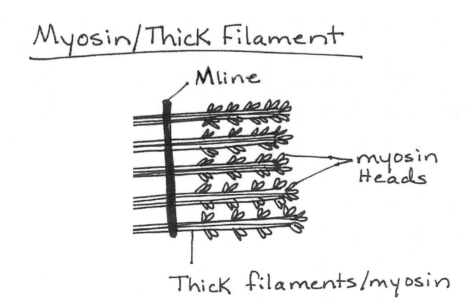

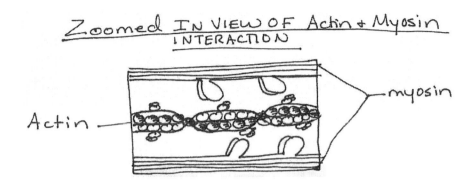

Zoomed IN VIEW OF Actin & Myosin INTERACTION

Actin —

— myosin

Sliding Filament Theory

During a contraction, every sarcomere's filaments slide along the myofibril. This will cause the myofibril to shorten, causing the muscle to shorten, which moves bones!

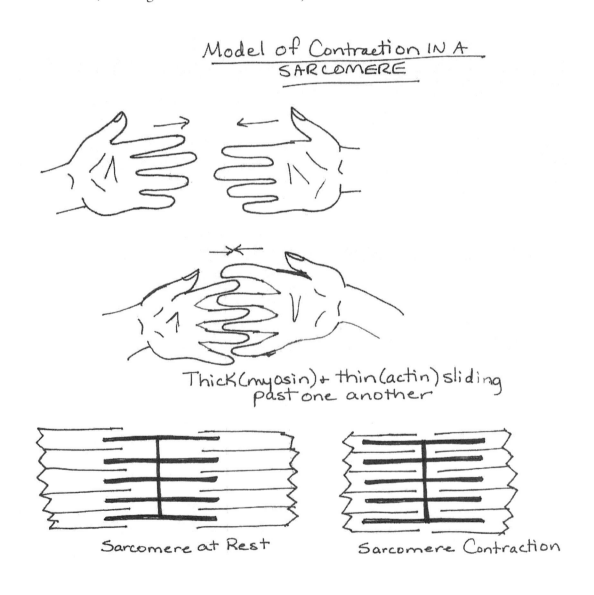

Model of Contraction IN A SARCOMERE

Thick (myosin) + thin (actin) sliding past one another

Sarcomere at Rest

Sarcomere Contraction

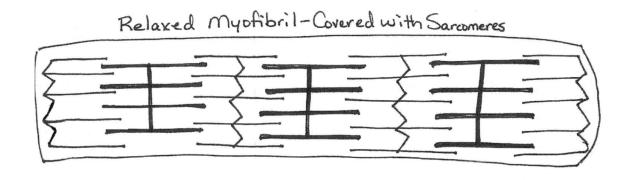

Relaxed Myofibril - Covered with Sarcomeres

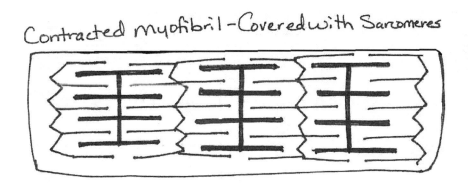

Contracted Myofibril - Covered with Sarcomeres

<u>Basics of a Neuron</u>

Muscle cells are under the control of the nervous system by cells called <u>neurons</u>. Neurons stimulate the sarcolemma of the muscle cell, in essence, telling the muscle to contract.

The area where the nervous system connects with the muscle fiber is called the <u>neuromuscular junction (NMJ)</u>. Each muscle fiber has one NMJ somewhere in the middle of its length. The <u>synaptic terminal</u> of the neuron is where the muscle fiber and neuron connect at the NMJ. The synaptic terminal has within it lots of vesicles that contain a <u>neurotransmitter</u> called <u>acetylcholine</u>. Huh? Well first we should know what the heck a neurotransmitter is! A neurotransmitter is a chemical messenger. Think about it this way, the brain cannot pop out of your skull and travel down to your toes to ask the muscles of your toes to wiggle, right? So how can the brain communicate with the muscles of the body without leaving the protection of the skull? Neurotransmitters! These are chemical messages that can tell the muscles when it is time to contract! Problem solved. Acetylcholine or ACh is a specific type of neurotransmitter that can help to change the permeability of another cell's plasma membrane. What does that mean? Don't worry, it will make sense in a bit! Stay with me! The ACh can help to trigger the muscle contraction, which is what we need to understand for now. Here's a more in depth set up of the NMJ:

Basics of A Neuron

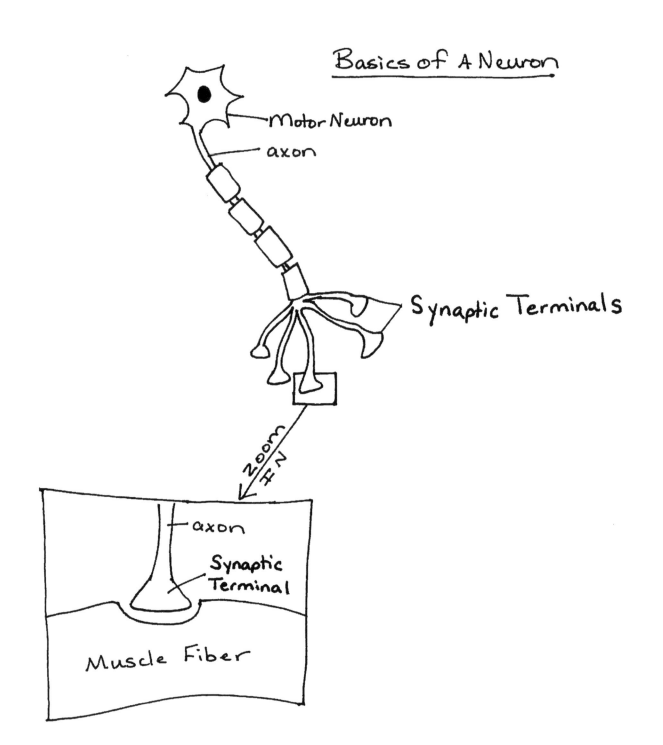

Motor Neuron

axon

Synaptic Terminals

Zoom #N

axon

Synaptic Terminal

Muscle Fiber

Neuromuscular Junction (NMJ)

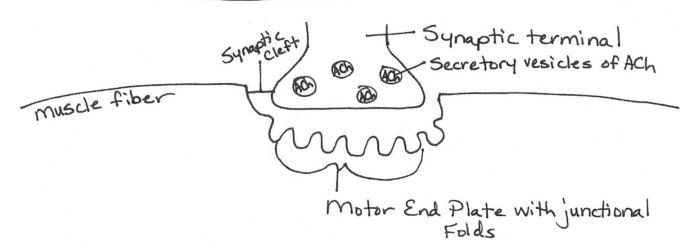

The <u>synaptic cleft</u> is the little space that is between the <u>synaptic terminal</u> and the muscle fiber. The surface of the muscle fiber below the <u>synaptic cleft</u> has receptors for binding ACh once it's released. This area containing receptors is called the <u>motor end plate</u>. The motor end plate has folds in it called <u>junctional folds</u> which increase the surface area so that more ACh can bind. We should also note that within the cleft is an enzyme called <u>acetylcholinesterase or AChE</u>. Acetylcholinesterase breaks down ACh so that the contraction can end.

Let's examine the steps of contraction.

An electrical impulse from the nervous system begins the process of contraction. We call this the <u>action potential</u>. Picture it as a little bolt of electricity. The action potential travels down through the axon to the synaptic terminal. When the action potential arrives at the terminal this will cause the ACh in the vesicles to be released by the process referred to as exocytosis (ejection from the cell). The ACh will spill into the cleft and bind to receptors on the sarcolemma's motor end plate. When the ACh binds to those receptors, this will make the sarcolemma more permeable to sodium or Na+. Remember from general bio that sodium is always present in extracellular fluid? Na+ will spill into the cytoplasm. This sudden rush of Na+ into the sarcoplasm will cause an action potential to form (remember the action potential is what will help this muscle fiber to start contraction). The action potential will travel through those T-tubules or highways leading through the cell. This action potential will cause the sarcoplasmic reticulum or SR to release calcium ions or Ca2+. The troponin/tropomyosin complex covers the active sites on the actin strand we previously introduced. Those active sites need to be exposed for contraction to occur. The Ca2+ will help with this! The Ca2+ binds to the troponin molecule which changes its shape and helps to roll the tropomyosin strand away from the active sites.

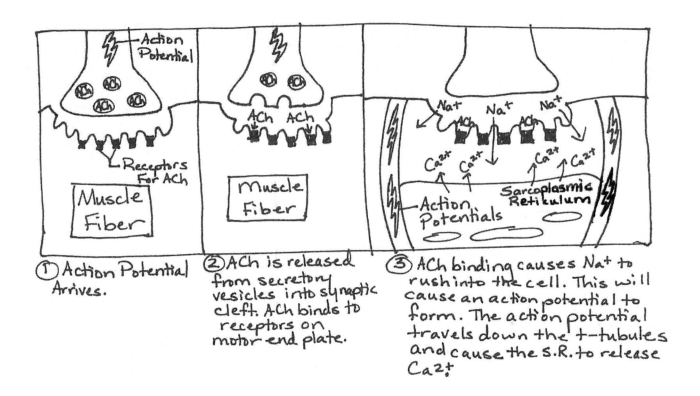

① Action Potential Arrives.

② ACh is released from secretory vesicles into synaptic cleft. ACh binds to receptors on motor end plate.

③ ACh binding causes Na+ to rush into the cell. This will cause an action potential to form. The action potential travels down the t-tubules and cause the S.R. to release Ca2+

The myosin heads of the myosin or thick filament are energized with ATP. Each myosin head has broken an ATP into ADP and phosphate and has stored the energy. When the myosin heads become energized this "cocks" the heads back. When the active sites previously mentioned are exposed, the energized myosin heads will bind to those active sites. The myosin heads joined to the actin strand are referred to as <u>cross-bridges</u>. After the cross-bridges form, the energy harnessed from ATP is released and the myosin head <u>power strokes</u> towards the M line. When another ATP binds to the myosin head this will cause the head to release from the active site and "cock" back again. As long as the active site is still exposed the head will bind again and power stroke again towards the M line.

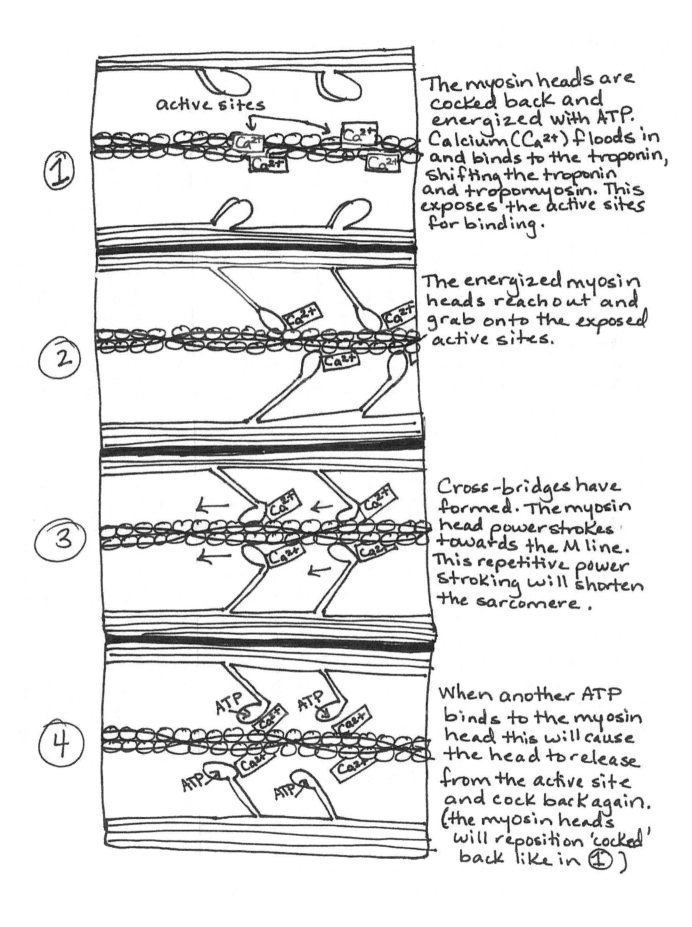

active sites

① The myosin heads are cocked back and energized with ATP. Calcium (Ca^{2+}) floods in and binds to the troponin, shifting the troponin and tropomyosin. This exposes the active sites for binding.

② The energized myosin heads reach out and grab onto the exposed active sites.

③ Cross-bridges have formed. The myosin head power strokes towards the M line. This repetitive power stroking will shorten the sarcomere.

④ When another ATP binds to the myosin head this will cause the head to release from the active site and cock back again. (the myosin heads will reposition 'cocked' back like in ①)

Imagine two men, each on opposite sides of a boat, pulling ropes with anchors towards the sides of the boat. The rope shortens and the anchors move closer to the center of the boat. The power strokes continue as contraction continues.

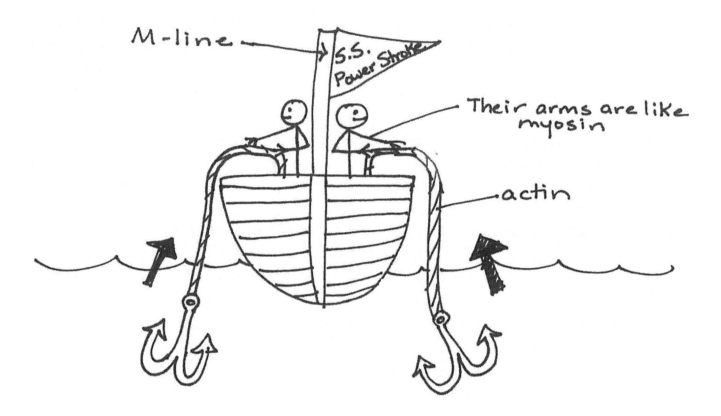

Motor Units

All of the muscle fibers controlled by one neuron is called a motor unit. One neuron can control hundreds of muscle fibers simultaneously.

Isotonic and Isometric Contractions

There are two main types of muscle contractions, isometric and isotonic. Isotonic contractions are when tension in the muscle increases and in addition the length of the muscle changes (like when you lift something up towards your chest and you see the muscle bulge). Isometric contractions are when the tension increases but the length of the muscle does not change. Like picking up a bucket of water and holding it by your side.

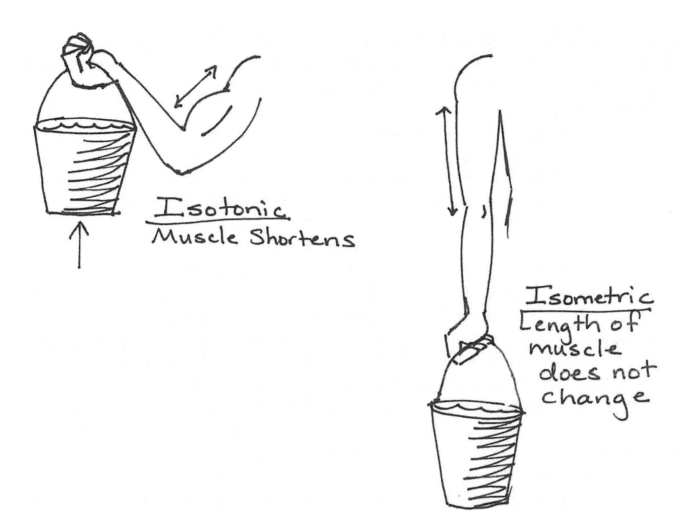

Isotonic
Muscle Shortens

Isometric
Length of muscle does not change

Types of Skeletal Muscle Fibers

Fast fibers contract quickly, have a large diameter and very few mitochondria. They are great at producing fast powerful contractions that don't last very long. These muscles tire quickly due to the limited amount of energy. Remember they have few mitochondria so it makes sense that they are not filled with abundant energy. Fast fibers tend to be pale in color as well and are often referred to as white muscle. This is like the white breast in a chicken or turkey.

Slow fibers are smaller than fast, take longer to stimulate, but have contractions that last much longer. Slow fibers are richer in blood supply and contain lots of mitochondria for an abundance of energy. Slow fibers also contain lots of myoglobin (which binds oxygen). Myoglobin is a red pigment and makes these fibers appear darker or red. This is what gives slow fibers the name red muscle. This is the same darker muscle we see in chicken and turkey legs (dark meat).

Intermediate fibers are most in appearance like fast fibers because they too are pale. They are more resistant against becoming tired in comparison to fast.

CHAPTER 11

Muscular System

A Flythrough to Complement Your Lab Study

NOTE: This chapter is to be read alongside your lab atlas/manual so that you may examine the muscles and structures for the lab portion of your course.

The arrangement of fascicles in a single muscle can greatly affect the strength and speed of motion in a contraction. In each fascicle the muscle fibers run parallel to each other, but in a muscle, the fascicles may run in different directions. Muscles can be grouped into categories based on fascicle arrangement:

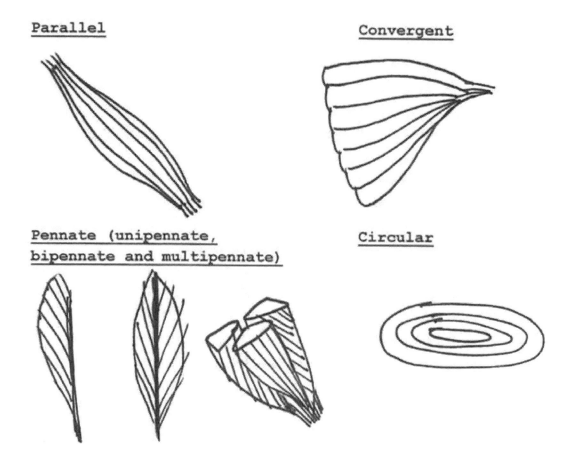

In a Parallel muscle the fascicles run in an organized parallel fashion. It's not just a clever name! Convergent muscles sort of look like a fan, the fascicles start out spread widely and converge or join together at a point (tendon). Pennate muscles typically form an angle with the tendon they are attached to. If the muscle has fibers only on one side of the tendon this would be called unipennate (picture half of a leaf). If there are fibers on both sides of the tendon this would be called bipennate (picture a whole leaf). If the tendon has branches in a pennate muscle this is called multipennate. Circular muscles, also known as sphincters, have fascicles in a circular pattern around an opening. These muscles are typically found around entrances and exits of the body as in the digestive tract.

Muscle Levers

Skeletal muscles are obviously attached to the skeleton, so where they attach can affect the strength and speed of the movement made in the muscle. In our bodies our bones act as levers for the skeletal muscles to work on. There are three main designations of levers. First class levers are like seesaws. Remember how fun those were?! The fulcrum is between the load and the force applied by the muscle. WHA?! Check this out…

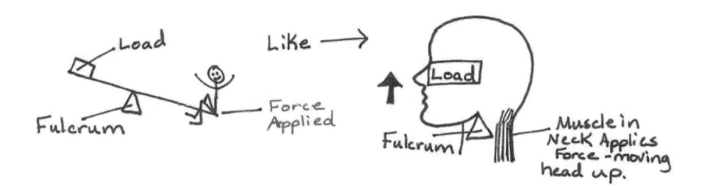

In Second class levers the load is between the fulcrum and the force applied by the muscle (kind of like a wheelbarrow).

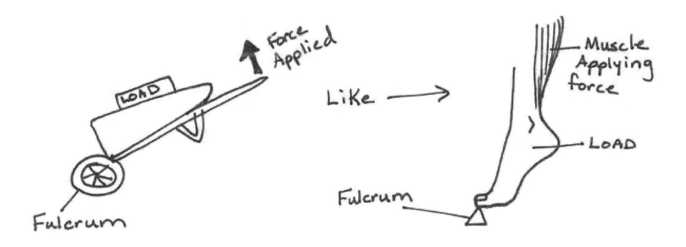

In <u>third class levers</u>, which are the most commonly found levers in the body, the force the muscle applies is between the load and the fulcrum.

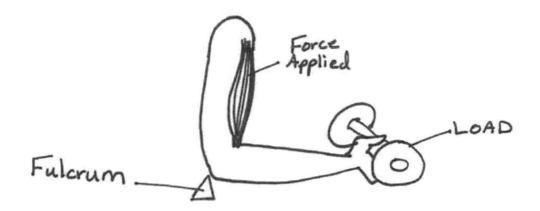

<u>Origin and Insertion</u>

Muscles typically have a moveable end and a stationary or non-moveable end. The moveable end of a muscle is called the <u>insertion</u>. This is the end that moves in a contraction towards the stationary end of the muscle. The stationary end is called the <u>origin</u>.

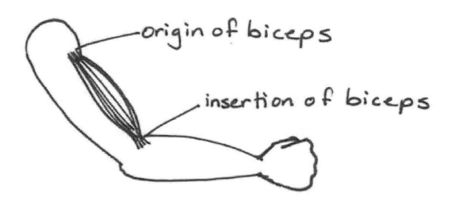

<u>Actions</u>

Skeletal muscle movements can include flexion, extension, rotation, abduction, adduction etc. (as previously covered in the articulation chapter). When we make movements with our muscles they typically work in groups. Based on what they do, muscles can be described in various ways. An <u>agonist</u> is a muscle that performs a prime movement, such as the bicep flexing the elbow. An <u>antagonist</u> is a muscle that produces an action that works against the agonist. An example would be the triceps extending the elbow. A <u>synergist</u> is a muscle that will assist the larger agonist so that it may work better. Finally, a <u>fixator</u> is a type of synergist that helps to stop or prevent movement at another joint and helps fix and support the origin of the agonist.

Axial and Appendicular Muscles

Axial Muscles are obviously found on the axial skeleton and will help to position the axis or center of the body. The appendicular muscles are found on the appendicular skeleton and will move the appendicular skeleton.

Please see your text/lab manual/atlas for study of the actual muscles and attachments

CHAPTER 12

Nervous Tissue

The nervous system is divided into two main parts, the <u>central nervous system (CNS)</u> and the <u>peripheral nervous system (PNS).</u> The CNS is central to the body and includes the brain and spinal cord. The CNS works to process and coordinate sensory information and motor commands. The sensory information could come from things you feel or detect outside the body (heat, wind blowing, a soft kiss on the cheek) or inside the body (gas pain, stomach ache, sore joint). The motor commands will cause an action, like the flexing of a muscle. I like to think of the sensory inputs as our "feelers" and the motor commands as our "doers." The CNS also is where our intelligence, memory and emotion lie. The PNS includes the nerves which carry sensory information into the CNS and motor commands out of the CNS. <u>Nerves</u> are bundles of axons. There are two types of nerves in the nervous system: <u>cranial nerves</u>, which are found connected to the brain, and <u>spinal nerves</u>, which are obviously connected to the...? You guessed it! The spine!

Remember how I previously mentioned that the sensory information comes into the CNS and the motor commands go out of the CNS? There's a name for that! The PNS can be further divided into the <u>afferent division</u> and the <u>efferent division</u>. The afferent division of the CNS will carry sensory information (from <u>receptors</u>) back to the CNS for processing. The efferent division will carry motor commands out of the CNS to areas of the body the CNS wants to activate (through <u>effectors</u> like the skeletal muscles).

The efferent division of the nervous system can be further broken down into two systems: The <u>somatic and autonomic nervous system.</u> The somatic nervous system or SNS specifically deals with the skeletal muscle contraction, or contractions that we choose to make. The autonomic nervous system or ANS helps with involuntary contraction of smooth muscle, cardiac muscle and glands. In other words, contractions or actions outside of your conscious control. So the ANS allows our heart to beat, our intestines and other digestive organs to contract and our glands to secrete. Thank goodness we aren't consciously in control of our heartbeat! The ANS includes a <u>sympathetic</u> and <u>parasympathetic division.</u> We will look into the sympathetic and parasympathetic divisions more closely in a later chapter.

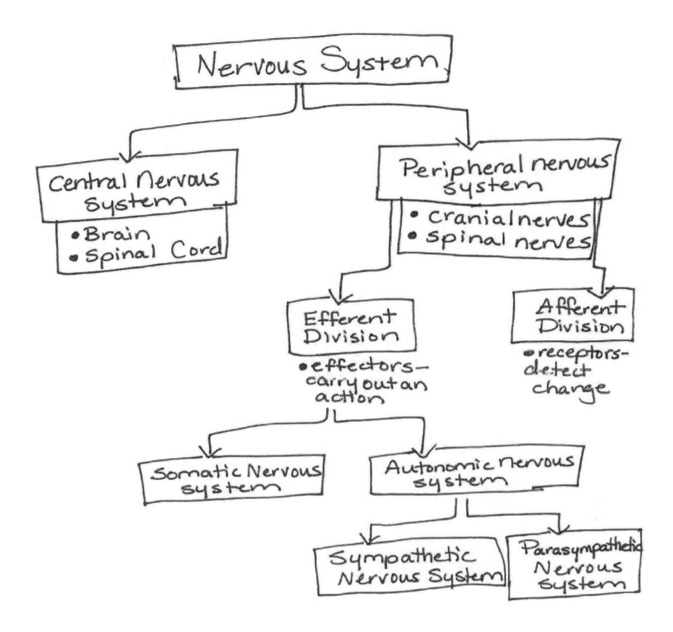

This chapter will focus primarily on the anatomy and function of the neuron. I'd like you to first think of the brain as the body's director. It gives commands to direct the organs and tissues of the body as well as interprets sensory information sent from the body to the brain. The brain is encased by the skull so obviously it can't step out of the skull and walk down to the hand to tell it to pick up a pencil. The brain needs to be able to talk to the body. It will do this through its electrical wiring or nerves. The nerves are like the electrical cords that lead from the electricity source to the appliance. The TV will only work if it is plugged in. The electricity moving through the cord powers the TV. This is similar to how the brain talks to the body. The nerves are like the cords connecting the appliances to the electricity source and the brain represents the electricity source. So the brain talks to the body through its wires—the nerves. The nerves are made up of cells called neurons. To understand how the brain talks to the body through nerves we must first understand the neuron.

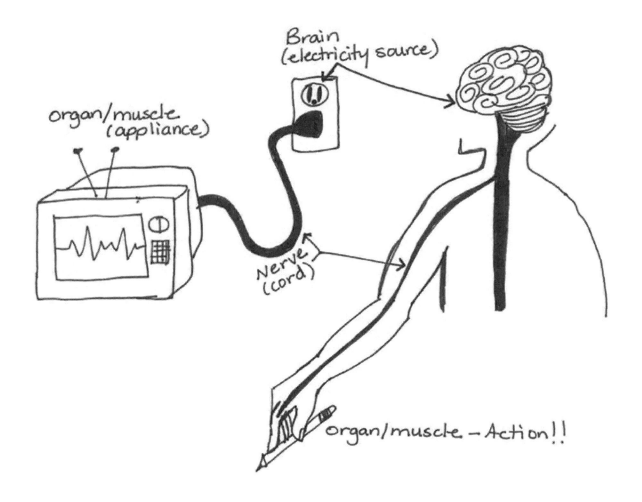

<u>Neurons</u>

The most common neuron in the CNS is called the <u>multipolar</u> neuron (pictured on the next page). This is the type of neuron we will focus on in our description. The neuron is made of several parts. The neuron has a large cell body. This is where the nucleus is found and a large portion of the cytoplasm called the <u>perikaryon</u>. The perikaryon has other organelles like the mitochondria for energy and the rough and smooth ER and ribosomes. The rough ER and ribosomes make protein. There are some areas in the cell body where rough ER and ribosomes are more numerous and gives the cell body a rough grainy appearance. Those areas are called <u>Nissl bodies</u>. They show up in close view as gray. This is where the term gray matter comes from. The cell body is covered with fine hair like processes called <u>dendrites.</u> Dendrites have many branches and can receive info from other neurons in the CNS. Coming off the cell body is a long process called the <u>axon</u>. The axon carries electrical impulses/action potentials. The axon is filled with cytoplasm called <u>axoplasm</u>. The axoplasm is covered in the axon by an <u>axolemma</u> or cell membrane. The first segment of the axon is called the <u>initial segment</u> which will be super important in the explanation about action potentials. The <u>axon hillock</u> is the thickened section of the axon coming off of the cell body. Sometimes axons branch, those branches are called <u>telodendria</u> which means tree. The telodendria end in synaptic <u>terminals</u> and are where the axons terminate/end.

The synaptic terminal is part of the knob-like ending of the neuron called the synapse. The synapse usually connects with another neuron or cell. When the synapse connects to another cell we call the first cell the presynaptic cell and the second cell the postsynaptic cell. There will be a gap between the pre and postsynaptic cell called the synaptic cleft.

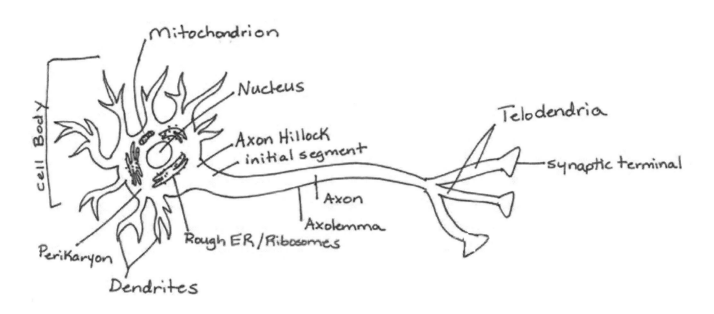

Other Types of Neurons

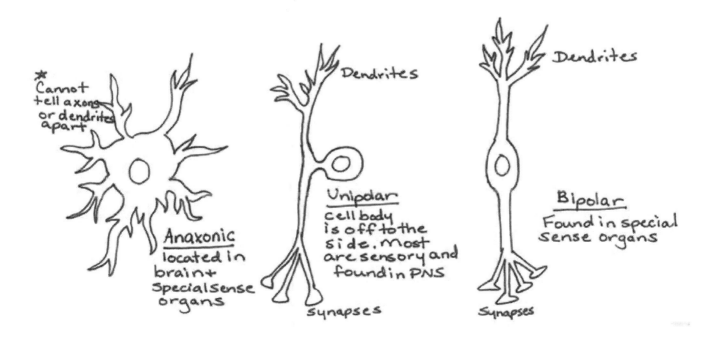

Presynaptic and Postsynaptic

The presynaptic cell usually sends a message to the postsynaptic cell through neurotransmitters. Remember we talked about neurotransmitters in the muscle chapter? They were the chemical messengers produced in the synapse that were released by secretory vesicles into the synaptic cleft for binding on the postsynaptic cell. Some presynaptic cells join with muscles like we talked about in chapter 10. That union is called a neuromuscular junction. A typical synaptic terminal is filled with organelles and vesicles of neurotransmitters. Neurotransmitters, once released, will be reabsorbed after they affect the postsynaptic cell. They are broken down and recycled at the synapse.

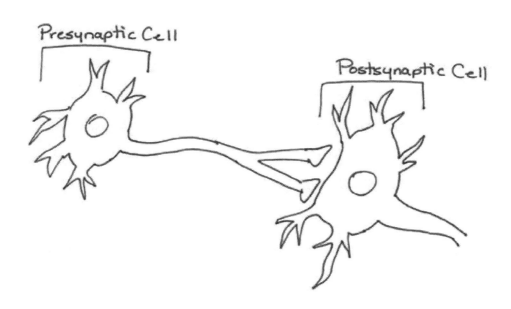

We noted the diversity in appearance of neurons but we can also separate neurons by function. Neurons can be <u>sensory, motor or interneurons</u>.

Sensory Neurons

Sensory neurons or afferent (coming into the CNS) bring info from the PNS into the CNS for processing. Sensory neurons are typically unipolar and connect a sensory receptor to the CNS. Sensory receptors can be <u>somatic or visceral</u>. The somatic sensory neurons keep us aware of our position in the outside world and the visceral sensory neurons make our bodies aware of our internal status. Sensory receptors can monitor our insides and outsides as mentioned above. The <u>interoceptors</u> (interior) monitor the majority of our internal systems: respiratory, urinary, digestive etc. The <u>exteroceptors</u> (exterior) give us information about our external surroundings: sight, smell, touch, temperature etc. <u>Propriocepters</u> interpret the position and movement of our joints and skeletal muscles.

Motor Neurons

Motor neurons or efferent neurons (coming out of the CNS) bring commands out of the CNS to the PNS for action. There are two types of motor neurons, somatic and visceral. The somatic motor neurons control skeletal muscles. The cell bodies of somatic motor neurons are found in the CNS. The axon of the somatic motor neuron runs in a peripheral nerve to the muscle tissue or neuromuscular junction. The visceral motor neurons are not under your conscious control and will help direct smooth and cardiac muscle, glands etc. in the body. There are visceral motor neurons in the CNS that connect with visceral motor neurons in the PNS. The set in the PNS are found in what is called the autonomic ganglia. <u>Ganglia</u> are collections of neuron cell bodies in the PNS. The set in the PNS ganglia are the ones that set the doers (effectors) into action.

Interneurons

Interneurons are primarily found in the CNS. Interneurons are typically found between sensory neurons and motor neurons. Their function is to hand out sensory information and direct motor commands. Interneurons also play a role in what are called our higher order (more fancy) functions like learning and memory.

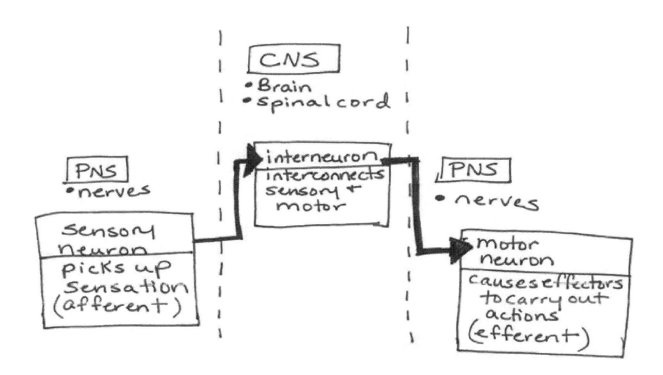

Neuroglia

Neuroglia are cells that protect the neurons and help them function properly. They are the glue that holds the neurons together. There are six types of neuroglia. Four are found in the CNS and two are found in the PNS. Let's begin with the CNS neuroglia.

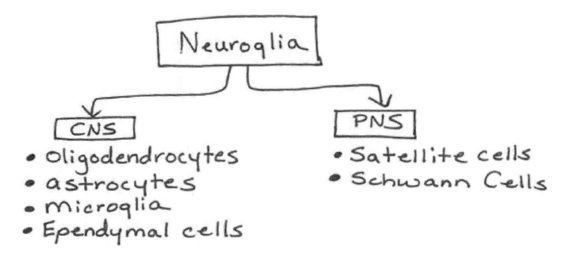

Oligodendrocytes are cells with many 'arms'. They wrap their arms around surrounding neurons. The arms wrap around the neuron forming a sort of insulation called the myelin sheath. I'll explain the usefulness of this insulation in a bit.

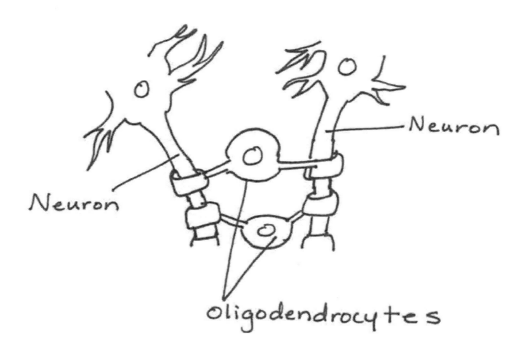

Astrocytes have a star-like shape and help to maintain the blood brain barrier (BBB) that works to control what is allowed to move from the main bloodstream into the brain tissue. They also help to recycle neurotransmitters.

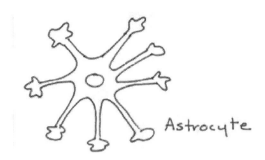

Ependymal Cells are found lining the ventricles of the brain and central canal of the spinal cord. They produce, circulate and monitor the cerebrospinal fluid (CSF). The CSF is found surrounding the brain and spinal cord and works to cushion and insulate CNS. The CSF also circulates nutrients and gases.

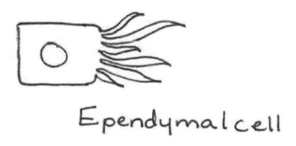

Microglia are types of macrophages that move around the CNS and phagocytize dead tissue, bacteria and any other substance that should not be in the CNS.

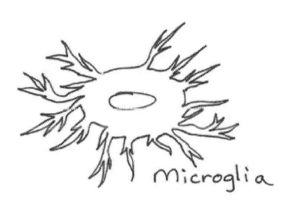

Schwann cells are found in the PNS and like the oligodendrocytes of the CNS, they insulate neurons in myelin sheaths.

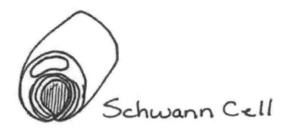

Satellite cells are also found in the PNS and surround cell bodies of the ganglia. They help to monitor neurotransmitter, oxygen and carbon dioxide levels in the ganglia.

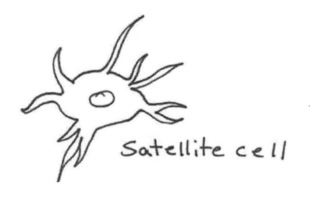

Myelin Sheath

The myelin sheath is an insulating sheath that covers the neuron like the rubber insulation found on a cord. Remember the TV cord drawing from before? The oligodendrocytes form this insulation in the CNS and the Schwann cells form them in the PNS. The oligodendrocytes have many arms, so they reach out and repeatedly wrap their arms around multiple neurons. This repeated wrapping forms insulation around the neurons. The myelination or insulation also makes the neurons appear white which is where the terminology 'white matter' comes from. It takes multiple oligodendrocytes to insulate an entire neuron. The Schwann cells wrap around a single nerve fiber. The insulated parts of a neuron are called the internodes whereas the non-insulated parts of a neuron are called the nodes or nodes of Ranvier.

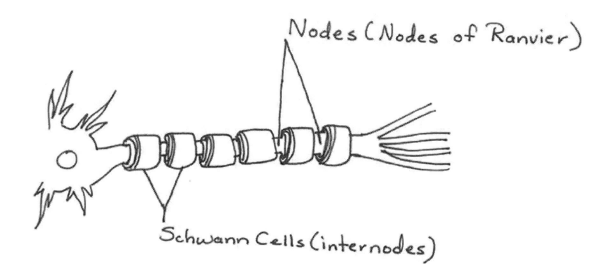

Nodes (Nodes of Ranvier)

Schwann Cells (internodes)

Not all neurons are myelinated. The neurons that are not myelinated in the CNS or PNS are called unmyelinated neurons. Unmyelinated neurons are not completely covered by neuroglia. Because they are not completely covered they appear darker and are referred to as <u>gray matter</u>. A myelinated neuron conducts impulses faster than an unmyelinated neuron. We will discuss why a bit later on in the chapter.

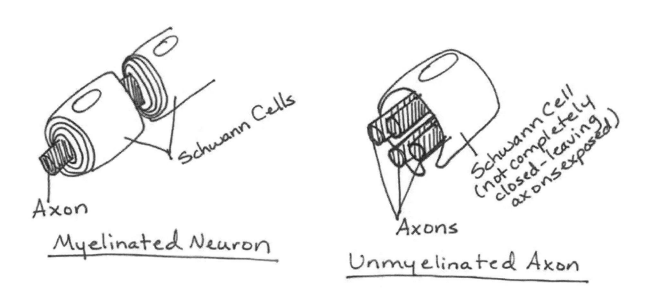

Schwann Cells

Axon

<u>Myelinated Neuron</u>

Schwann Cell (not completely closed—leaving axons exposed)

Axons

<u>Unmyelinated Axon</u>

Electrical or Transmembrane Potential

In order for neurons to talk to one another or talk to tissues they use electrical potentials and currents—like the current in electrical wiring. The <u>transmembrane potential</u> is defined as the difference in electrical potential across a membrane. The <u>resting membrane potential</u> is the transmembrane potential in a resting cell. The resting membrane potential of the neuron is about -70mV (millivolts). The negative sign in front of the 70 means that there are more negatively charged particles on the inside of the cell than the outside. Electrical currents in the body are made by the charged ions that flow in and out of cells such as Na+ (sodium) and K+ (potassium). There are channels that allow these ions to flow in and out. The body can control these channels to turn that flow off or on. That ability will be beneficial for the 'firing' of neurons. In a resting cell there is an uneven distribution of charged ions/molecules between the inside of the cell and the outside of the cell. The sodium and potassium play the largest role in this difference. There is more K+ on the inside of the cell than the outside. K+ will flow down its concentration gradient through leak channels, meaning it will flow from a high concentration to a low concentration. K+ will flow naturally out of the cell. Na+ is much higher on the outside of the cell membrane, so it too will flow down its concentration gradient through leak channels or from the outside of the cell to the inside. A type of gated channel called the sodium potassium pump in the cell membrane will help to balance this leakage of ions. Gated channels will open or close in response to stimuli. The sodium potassium pump will pump three Na+ out of the cell for every two K+ it brings into the cell. This exchange will keep the resting membrane potential of -70mV.

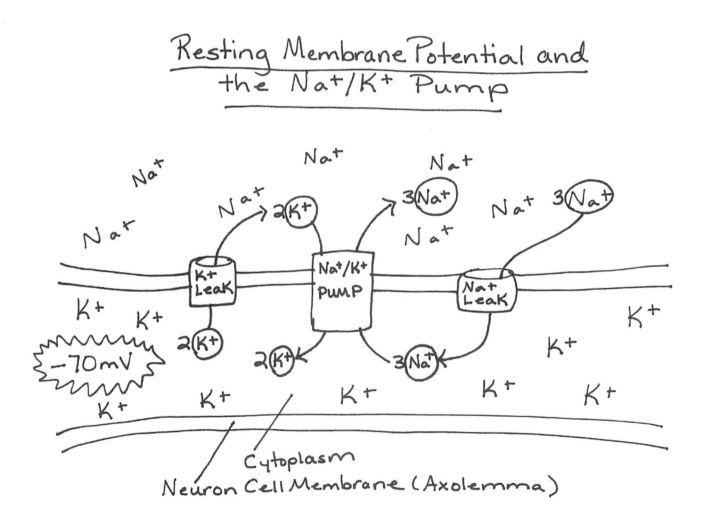

If a transmembrane potential is disturbed in a neuron, the neuron 'fires.' Light, heat and chemicals can cause stimulation of a neuron. When a neuron is at rest most gated channels are closed. If those gated channels were to open, ions could rush in or out of the cell and change the transmembrane potential. Graded potentials are changes in the transmembrane potential that are localized.

Action Potentials

In order for a neuron to 'fire,' an action potential must take place. An action potential is a change caused by the opening of voltage-gated ion channels. Voltage-gated ion channels open or close in response to changes in transmembrane potential. Action potentials cause a dramatic up and down of transmembrane potential.

Steps of the Action Potential

1) Na+ will rush into the neuron at the axon hillock, depolarizing it. **Remember from chapter 10 that depolarization means to change the transmembrane potential towards a less negative number.** This is a local potential meaning a change at this specific spot on the neuron. This change needs to spread to fully stimulate the neuron.

2) For the stimulus to spread we must reach threshold (-55 mV). If we reach this number the other voltage-gated ion channels will open causing the impulse to spread. Once -55 mV is reached the neuron will 'fire.' The Na+ and K+ channels will open. Na+ will rush into the cell which will further drive the transmembrane potential towards a less negative number (depolarization). As the rising transmembrane potential creeps towards 0 mV, Na+ channels begin to close. Once they have all closed the cell's transmembrane potential will be about +35 mV.

3) Now the K+ gates will be fully opened and K+ will rush out of the cell, repolarizing the cell. **Remember from chapter 10 repolarization means to change the transmembrane potential back towards negative numbers.** K+ gates stay open a bit too long causing the transmembrane potential to go past the resting membrane potential rate of -70 mV. This is called hyperpolarization.

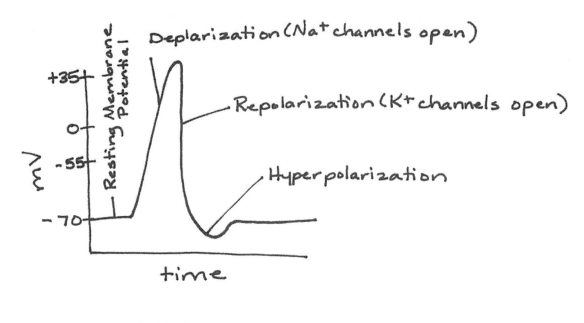

Action Potential

The Refractory Period

The refractory period is the period of time that it is either very difficult or impossible to stimulate the neuron. There are two major types of refractory periods: absolute refractory periods and relative refractory periods. In the absolute refractory period, no amount of stimulation will start a new action potential. The absolute refractory period lasts the duration of the action potential until the cell reaches resting membrane potential again after repolarization. In the relative refractory period it would be possible to stimulate the neuron, but only with an extremely strong stimulus. The relative refractory period lasts the duration of the hyperpolarization phase.

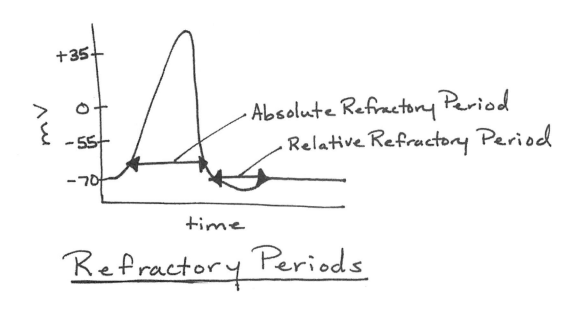

Refractory Periods

Propagation of Action Potentials

Action potentials must spread along the axon membrane, meaning, the entire axon needs to know what is going on. It's not good enough that the initially stimulated segment has been depolarized, the whole axon should be stimulated so that eventually the synaptic terminal can release a neurotransmitter. Propagation of an action potential refers to each segment of an axon repeating the message (action potential) over and over. There are two main types of propagation to cover, continuous propagation and saltatory propagation.

Continuous propagation will occur in an unmyelinated axon. Imagine for simplicity that the axon is divided into segments (numbered in the illustration below). The action potential will start at the initial segment. The membrane will depolarize to +30mV. The sodium ions from the depolarization in the initial segment will spread away from the open channel (local current) which will began to bring the membrane of segment 2 to threshold. Segment 2 will now complete depolarization while segment 1 starts to repolarize. Similarly as segment 2 has depolarized, sodium ions will sweep forward towards segment 3 causing it to reach threshold while segment 2 begins to repolarize towards refractory. This will continue until we reach the end of the axon.

When a local current develops the action potential can only move forward because the segment previous is in the refractory period. This will ensure that the action potential always moves in a forward direction.

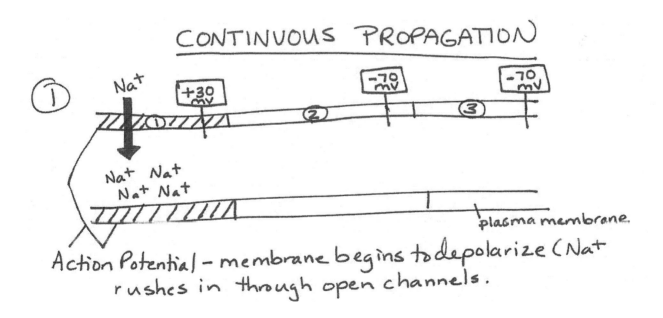

- 75 -

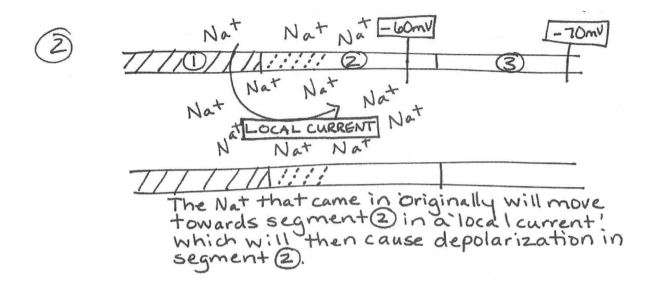

The Na⁺ that came in originally will move towards segment ② in a local current! which will then cause depolarization in segment ②.

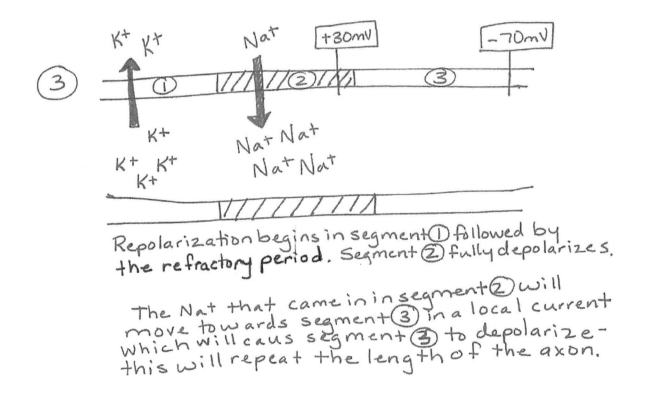

Repolarization begins in segment ① followed by the refractory period. Segment ② fully depolarizes.

The Na⁺ that came in in segment ② will move towards segment ③ in a local current which will caus segment ③ to depolarize- this will repeat the length of the axon.

Saltatory propagation occurs in myelinated neurons. This type of propagation occurs much faster than continuous propagation. Recall the illustration of the myelinated neuron and the areas on it labeled nodes or internodes. Saltatory propagation only has to depolarize the nodes of the axon 'jumping' over the internodes of the axon.

The action potential will occur at the initial segment. A local current of sodium will be produced and sweep forward to the next node where it will bring this node to threshold. The second node will depolarize, the local current will sweep forward to node 3 which will enter threshold. Node two begins to enter the refractory period. Due to the myelin insulation only the nodes will respond to a stimulus allowing us to skip the stimulation of the internode portions of the axon. WAY FASTER! WAY AWESOME!

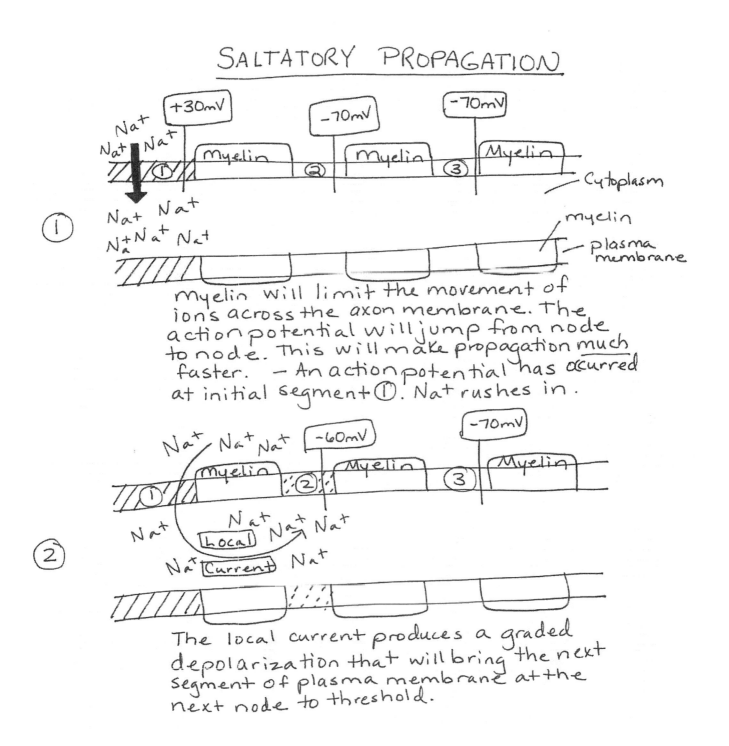

SALTATORY PROPAGATION

myelin will limit the movement of ions across the axon membrane. The action potential will jump from node to node. This will make propagation much faster. — An action potential has occurred at initial segment①. Na⁺ rushes in.

The local current produces a graded depolarization that will bring the next segment of plasma membrane at the next node to threshold.

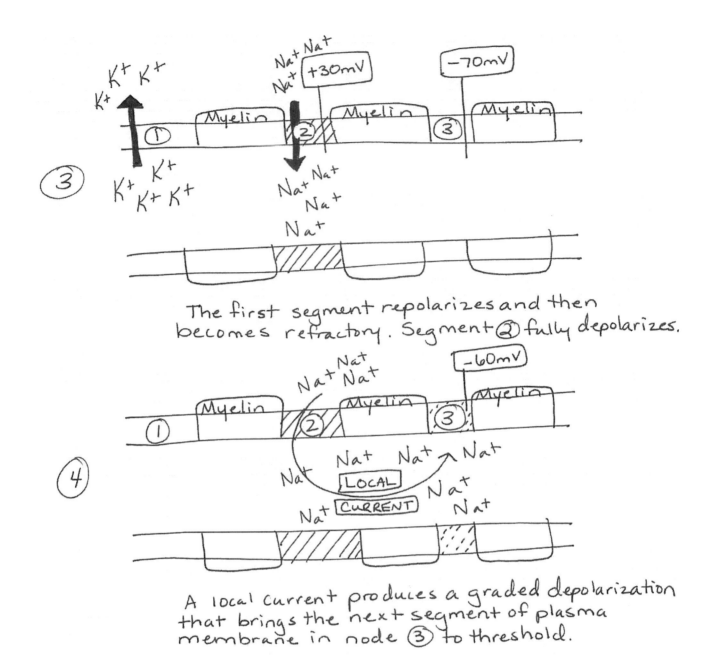

The first segment repolarizes and then becomes refractory. Segment ② fully depolarizes.

A local current produces a graded depolarization that brings the next segment of plasma membrane in node ③ to threshold.

Remember the point of all this? Relaying a message? Now that we understand the movement of an action potential, what happens next?

Synaptic activity is what!!!

At synapses there will be communication between fellow neurons or between neurons and other cells. When we have communication or conversation between two neurons we can label the neurons as <u>presynaptic</u> or <u>postsynaptic</u>. A presynaptic neuron is one who does all the 'talking' and the post-synaptic neuron is one who does all the 'listening' or receives the message. Synapses can be classi-fied or grouped into electrical or chemical synapses. Let's talk electrical first.

In electrical synapses the pre and postsynaptic membranes will actually touch together at gap junctions. Remember those? Those were the tiny little pores that allowed ions to flow back and forth between cells. In this close relationship if one neuron is being stimulated and is propagating an action potential, that stimulus will spread to the postsynaptic cell too.

In chemical synapses, which are much more common, the pre and postsynaptic neurons do not contact each other and therefore must use chemicals to 'talk.' The chemicals used are called neurotransmitters. Remember acetylcholine or ACh? Yeah, it's back to haunt us. It is a neurotransmitter. Neurotransmitters can be excitatory or inhibitory. Excitatory would stimulate a neuron to propagate action potentials where an inhibitory would discourage the formation and propagation of action potentials.

Cholinergic synapses are synapses that release our friend acetylcholine (Ach).

CHAPTER 13

<u>Spinal Cord and Nerves</u>

<u>A Flythrough to Complement Your Lab Study</u>

NOTE: This chapter is to be read alongside your lab atlas/manual so that you may examine the nerves and structures for the lab portion of your course.

The brain cannot leave the skull and march down to the hands to tell them to pick up a pencil right? RIGHT! The brain must be able to 'talk' to the rest of the body without leaving the comfort and protection of the skull. The nervous system uses the nerves for this task. They get things done! The brain and spinal cord make up the central nervous system or CNS, remember? The cranial and spinal nerves make up the peripheral nervous system or PNS. The PNS will work on reflexes. Reflexes are automatic responses to stimuli. A spinal reflex can be handled entirely by the spinal cord with no involvement from the brain at all. If you walked into the kitchen and rested your hand on the hot stove not knowing it was recently turned on, you would jerk your hand back to avoid further pain before your brain even knew anything happened.

<u>Organization of the Spinal Cord</u>

The adult spinal cord is about 45 cm long and about 14mm wide. The spinal cord does not reach the end of the vertebral column and instead ends between the vertebrae L1 and L2. On the posterior surface of the spinal cord there is a shallow groove called the <u>posterior median sulcus</u>. Similarly on the anterior side there is a deeper groove called the <u>anterior median fissure.</u> The spinal cord, like the brain, is made of gray and white matter. The amount of gray matter is greatest in parts of the spinal cord that are primarily responsible for sensory and motor command of the limbs. The cervical enlargement is an area that supplies nerves to the shoulder and upper limbs where the lumbar enlargement helps control the pelvis and lower limbs. Below the lumbar enlargement the spinal cord becomes skinnier and is called the <u>conus medullaris</u>. The <u>filum terminale</u> is a very skinny strand of tissue that extends from the tip of the conus medullaris. (See textbook for anatomy) The spinal cord is divided into 31 segments based on where the spinal nerves originate. Each segment is lettered and numbered similar to the vertebrae. Every spinal segment is associated with a pair of <u>dorsal root ganglia</u> close to the spinal cord. This is where the cell bodies of sensory neurons are found. The axons of those neurons form the <u>dorsal roots</u>. The dorsal roots are what bring the sensory information to the spinal cord. Conversely, the <u>ventral roots</u> contain the axons of motor neurons that will help control somatic and visceral effectors. (Remember what those terms mean from chapter 12?) The sensory and motor nerves will be stuck together into a spinal nerve which is mixed—that means they have both sensory and motor fibers. Cool huh? There are 31 pairs of spinal nerves.

The vertebral column is surrounded by a fantastic set of shock absorbers called the <u>spinal meninges</u>. These guys are so fancy they also contain a series of blood vessels that branch in them to deliver oxygen and nutrients to the spinal cord. There are three layers of meninges that also mirror the meningeal layers of the brain. The three meninges are <u>1) dura mater, 2) arachnoid mater, and 3) pia mater.</u>

The <u>dura mater</u> is super tough and fibrous. It forms the outermost covering of the cord. It has plentiful amounts of collagen to give it extra elasticity.

The <u>arachnoid mater</u> is the middle meningeal layer. It also contains lots of collagen and elastic fibers.

The <u>pia mater</u> is the innermost meningeal layer and has blood vessels that feed the spinal cord running along it.

The anatomy of the spinal nerves and their organization is best viewed in your text. See you in chapter 14 for brain talk!

CHAPTER 14

The Brain and Cranial Nerves

A Flythrough to Complement Your Lab Study

NOTE: This chapter is to be read alongside your lab atlas/manual so that you may examine the brain and nerves for the lab portion of your course.

The adult human brain contains about 97 percent of the body's neural tissue. We will discuss the anatomical organization of the brain and the function of its main parts in this chapter. The major brain regions are: the cerebrum, cerebellum, diencephalon, midbrain, pons, and medulla oblongata. The largest part of the brain is the cerebrum which is divided into right and left cerebral hemispheres. The brain is also covered in a cortex which is a thin layer of gray matter. The surface of the brain as you have likely noticed is very bumpy and folded. Those folds and bumps have names. The deep grooves or crevices are called fissures, the shallow grooves are called sulci and the elevated 'wormy' bumps are called gyri. Some MAJOR stuff happens in the cerebrum. This is where most higher mental functions happen. The cerebellum is the second largest part of the brain and it too is divided into hemispheres and is covered by a cortex. The cerebellum is pretty important too—if you consider being able to perform major movements important.

If we remove the cerebral and cerebellar hemispheres we can then better see the diencephalon. The diencephalon is made of the thalamus (left and right) and the hypothalamus. The thalamus will bring in sensory information and help to process it. The hypothalamus makes up the bottom of the diencephalon. It will help with emotions, hormone function and autonomic function. (The pituitary gland buds off of the hypothalamus—but we'll save that for a later chapter). The diencephalon links the hemispheres of the cerebrum and the brain stem. The brain stem is SUPER important! It will process info headed to and from the cerebrum and cerebellum. The brain stem includes the mesencephalon, pons, and medulla oblongata. The mesencephalon will process what you see and hear and control the reflexes that will be triggered by those stimuli. The pons connects the cerebellum to the brain stem and is involved in somatic and visceral motor control. The medulla oblongata connects the brain and spinal cord. It will help to regulate functions like heart rate, blood pressure and digestion.

So, since the brain is so critical to all life's functions it must be super well protected right? Right! It is protected by the skull, three meningeal layers, the cerebrospinal fluid (CSF), and the blood brain barrier or BBB.

THE 'MAIN BRAIN'

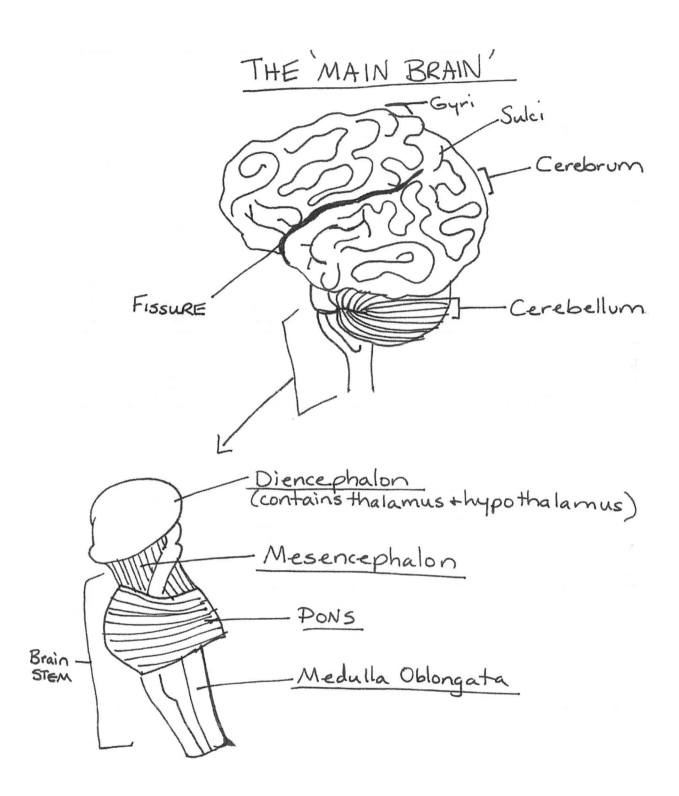

Gyri

Sulci

Cerebrum

Fissure

Cerebellum

Diencephalon
(contains thalamus + hypothalamus)

Mesencephalon

Pons

Brain STEM

Medulla Oblongata

The cranial meninges are the same three discussed in the last chapter. The dura mater, arachnoid mater and pia mater. The dura mater is made of an outer and inner fibrous layer. The outer layer is actually fused to the periosteum of the cranial bones. The outer and inner meningeal layers of the dura mater are separated by a space that contains tissue fluids and blood vessels. The arachnoid mater is made of the arachnoid membrane and the cells and fibers of the arachnoid trabeculae that cross the subarachnoid space to the pia mater. The pia mater sticks to the surface of the brain and is held down by the astrocytes we mentioned previously.

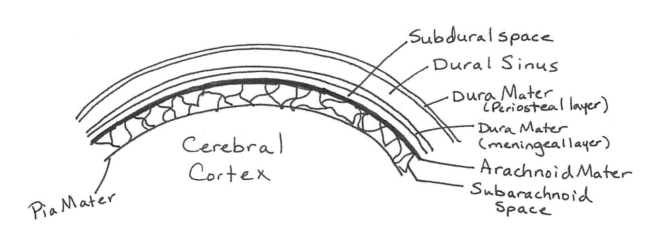

CRANIAL MENINGES

The dural folds are areas where the dura mater stretches into the cranial cavity. These dural folds will give the brain additional support and stability.

The cerebrospinal fluid or CSF completely surrounds and bathes the CNS. It will support the brain, cushion it from shock, deliver nutrients and transport chemical messengers and waste products. The choroid plexus is an area in each ventricle that produces CSF. Ependymal cells that have microvilli are connected by tight junctions and surround the capillaries of the choroid plexus. They will secrete CSF into the ventricles and also remove waste from the CSF. WOW!

Since the brain requires a lot of oxygen and nutrients it has to have a constant blood supply. This is achieved by the carotid arteries and the vertebral arteries. Blood will leave the brain via the jugular veins. Neural tissue in the CNS is separated from the general circulation by the blood brain barrier or BBB. The BBB consists of the endothelial capillary cells that are interconnected by tight junctions. Tight junctions will not allow material to diffuse between endothelial cells. The things that can diffuse across the membrane are lipid soluble and would include oxygen, carbon dioxide, ammonia, lipids (steroids or prostaglandins) and small alcohols. These things can diffuse into the interstitial fluid of the brain and spinal cord. The water and ions must pass through the apical and basement plasma membranes whereas larger compounds can cross the capillary walls only by active or passive transport. The astrocytes previously mentioned play a role in how restrictive permeability is in the endothelial lining of the capillaries. They will release chemicals that will control how permeable the endothelium will be to various substances. Transport of substances across the BBB is selective. All ions are controlled (Na+, H+, Cl-, K+). Neurons are in constant need of glucose to function no matter what the levels are in the rest of the body. Endothelial cells always allow a free pass to glucose.

Medulla Oblongata

The medulla oblongata is the most inferior of the brain regions. It is a very busy part of the brain. The brain and spinal cord communicate through the medulla oblongata through tracts that descend through it. It is also a center for coordinating complex autonomic reflexes and control of visceral functions. The medulla oblongata contains two main reflex centers: the cardiovascular center and respiratory rhythmicity center. The cardiovascular center will regulate the heart rate and force of contraction and the respiratory rhythmicity center will set the pace of respiratory movements. Please see book for anatomy of nerves etc.

Pons

The pons links the cerebellum with the midbrain, diencephalon, cerebrum, and spinal cord. It contains nuclei and tracts that carry sensory and motor information. Please see book for anatomy of nerves etc.

Cerebellum

The cerebellum is an automatic processing center and will do two main things. 1) it will work to adjust the posture muscles of the body to help keep balance. It will do this by modifying motor centers in the brain stem. 2) It will program and fine tune movements controlled at the conscious and subconscious levels. It will refine learned movements by regulating activity along motor pathways at the cerebral cortex and brain stem. In other words it smoothes your movements out! Please see your book for anatomy etc.

The Midbrain

The midbrain's main functions are to integrate visual information with other sensory input. In other words it will allow you to respond to visual stimuli with reflex responses. It will also relay auditory info to allow you to respond to auditory stimuli with reflex responses. (ex. A loud unexpected noise causes your body to jump involuntarily) It will also allow you to maintain posture and body position, and will assist in maintaining consciousness and alertness. Please see your book for anatomy etc.

The Diencephalon

The diencephalon is made of the epithalamus, thalamus and hypothalamus. The epithalamus contains the pineal gland which secretes melatonin to help regulate the day and night cycle. The thalamus contains part of the limbic system which deals with emotions. It will also project sensory information to the frontal lobes, relay information to the motor area of cerebral cortex from cerebellum, integrate sensory info for projection to areas of cerebral cortex, project visual info to the visual cortex, auditory info to auditory cortex and integrate sensory info and influence emotional state. (I'm pretty sure that part of me is overactive!) Please see your book for anatomy etc. The hypothalamus secretes <u>oxytocin</u> to stimulate smooth muscle contractions in the uterus and stimulates active mammary glands to release milk. The hypothalamus regulates body temp by controlling autonomic centers in medulla oblongata, controls heart rate and blood pressure by regulation of autonomic centers in the medulla oblongata. It will produces hormones that inhibit or stimulate endocrine cells of the anterior lobe of the pituitary gland. It also controls feeding reflexes (swallowing etc.), regulates circadian rhythm, and secretes antidiuretic hormone or ADH which will restrict water loss by the kidneys. Are you tired yet?? Please see book for anatomy etc.

The Limbic System

The limbic system is a grouping of nuclei and tracts along the border between the cerebrum and diencephalon. The limbic system is responsible for linking the conscious intellectual functions of the cerebral cortex with the unconscious and autonomic functions of the brain stem. It will establish emotional states and will control memory storage and retrieval of those memories. The limbic system makes you want to complete tasks, therefore it is sometimes referred to as the motivational system.

The Cerebrum

The cerebrum is the largest region of the brain and will contain sensory, motor and association areas. This is where your conscious thoughts and all high order intellectual functions originate. The cerebrum does a lot of work in processing somatic, sensory and motor information.

The cerebral cortex is a layer on the outside of the brain that covers the two cerebral hemispheres and measures in a range from about 1-4.5 mm thick. Each hemisphere receives sensory info from and sends motor commands to, the opposite side of the body. Meaning the left hemisphere controls muscles on the right side of the body and vice versa. The inside of the cerebrum consists mostly of white matter. The axons of white can be classified as <u>association fibers, commissural fibers and projection fibers</u>. Association fibers interconnect areas of the cerebral cortex inside of a single cerebral hemisphere. Commissural fibers interconnect and allow communication between the hemispheres. Projection fibers connect the cerebral cortex to the diencephalon, brain stem, cerebellum and spinal cord. Please examine your text for anatomy of the fibers and how they run along the brain.

As your cerebral cortex consciously directs complex problem solving of puzzles or complex movements, there are other areas of the brain that are processing sensory information and motor commands outside of your awareness. A lot of these activities are directed by the <u>basal nuclei</u>. The basal nuclei are masses of gray matter that are deep to the floor of the lateral ventricle in each hemisphere. They are found surrounded by white matter. The basal nuclei include the <u>caudate nucleus, lentiform nucleus, claustrum and amygdaloid body</u>. The caudate nucleus and lentiform nucleus function in subconscious adjustment of voluntary motor commands. The claustrum is primarily responsible for the subconscious processing of visual info and the amygdaloid body is a component of the limbic system. See your book for anatomy of the basal nuclei.

An electroencephalogram or EEG is a printed recording of the electrical activity of the brain or brain waves. Alpha waves are a characteristic waves found in normal resting adults. Beta waves are recorded when someone is concentrating intensely. Theta waves are seen in children and agitated adults. Delta waves are found in deep sleep. See your text for detail on cranial reflexes and the anatomy of cranial nerves.

CHAPTER 15

<u>Sensory Pathways and the Somatic Nervous System</u>

<u>A Flythrough to Complement Your Lab Study</u>

NOTE: This chapter is to be read alongside your lab atlas/manual so that you may examine the somatic pathways and somatic nervous system for the lab portion of your course.

Now that we have the physiology of neurons down and the major landmarks of the brain and spinal cord we can start to discuss how the nervous system parts work together. Remember that sensory information is what we gather inside our bodies or from our outside world. This includes the stimuli that we see, hear, taste or feel around us. All sensory information must be routed to the brain for processing. More specifically, it must be routed to the <u>somatosensory cortex</u> of the brain for processing. Recall that sensory receptors are specialized cells or processes that monitor specific conditions in the body or external environment. The receptors must pass info to our CNS in the form of action potentials along the axon of a sensory neuron. The nerves and tracts that deliver somatic and visceral info to the brain are called the <u>sensory pathways</u>. The receptors, sensory neurons and pathways are part of the afferent division. Somatic info is carried to sensory processing centers in the brain, typically the <u>primary sensory cortex </u>of the cerebrum, or appropriate areas of the cerebellum. We will also discuss the somatic motor part of the efferent division that includes the tracts and motor neurons that control peripheral effectors. Whether the motor commands are conscious or subconscious they will still travel along the somatic motor pathways that control skeletal muscles. The motor neurons and pathways that control the skeletal muscles are called the <u>somatic nervous system or SNS</u>.

Sensory receptors are designed to connect our internal and external environment with our nervous system. Remember that sensory receptors are cells that will give your CNS info about what is going on inside and outside your body. This could include temperature, pain, vibration, body position or touch. The CNS will interpret the information on the basis of the frequency of the action potentials arriving at any particular time. When pressure sensations are arriving, the harder the pressure, the higher the frequency of action potentials. This information is called a <u>sensation</u>. When you are aware of a sensation we call this a <u>perception</u>. The special senses are: <u>olfaction</u> (fancy word for smell), <u>vision</u>, <u>gustation</u> (fancy for taste), <u>balance or equilibrium</u> and <u>hearing</u>. The special sense receptors are more complicated and are called the <u>sense organs</u> (eye or ear for example). We'll discuss these in chapter 17. When a sensory receptor picks up on a stimulus it will translate that stimulus to the CNS via an action potential. This translation is called <u>transduction</u>.

In order for any of this to happen, the receptor must detect the stimulus in the first place. How does this happen? Each receptor has a characteristic sensitivity. A touch receptor would be very sensitive to pressure but insensitive to chemical stimuli. Conversely, a taste bud would be sensitive to chemicals in food but not sensitive to pressure. This is called receptor specificity. This specificity may come from the receptor's structure or the presence of accessory cells that block the receptor from other types of stimuli. The simplest type of receptors are called free nerve endings. These are sensory neurons with branched dendrites that extend through tissue like the branches of a root system. These receptors are open to many different types of stimuli, meaning they don't show much receptor specificity. The area under the control of a specific receptor cell is its receptor field. If a stimulus occurs in the receptor field, the CNS will receive the information as a stimulus received from a specific receptor. If the stimulus occurs across a large area it may be more difficult to localize the stimulus to a particular area. A stimulus can come in many forms: chemical, touch, sound, or light. The transduction of a stimulus into an action potential begins when the stimulus changes the membrane potential of a receptor cell (receptor potential). A receptor potential is either a graded depolarization or a graded hyperpolarization (chapter 12). The stronger a stimulus is, the larger the receptor potential. The receptors for the general senses are usually the dendrites of the sensory neurons. If there is a depolarizing receptor potential in a neural receptor, we call this a generator potential.

Sensory information must be routed once it arrives at the CNS. This routing will occur based on the location and type of stimulus. If the sensation is touch, the sensation must travel along sensory pathways to the region of the cerebral cortex designed to interpret it. The connection between the peripheral receptor and the cortical neuron is called a labeled line. The labeled line is made of axons that carry info about one type of stimulus (ex. touch). The CNS will interpret the type of stimulus it is by which labeled line it crossed. If the stimulus crosses the labeled line of touch, the CNS knows the sensation is touch. Isn't that amazing?! Where the sensory info arrives in the sensory cortex of the brain will help the brain determine the location of the stimulus. For example, if the activity is in a labeled line region that carries touch sensations that stimulate the facial region of the primary sensory cortex, we perceive we are being touched on our face. The strength of the stimulus as mentioned before is determined by the frequency and pattern of the arriving action potentials.

Some sensory neurons are called tonic receptors because they are always active. Other receptors are called phasic receptors and are not usually active. The phasic receptors can provide info about how intense a stimulus is or its rate of change. The receptors that combine phasic and tonic coding are the ones that convey complicated sensory info.

Adaptation is a reduced sensitivity to a constant, repeating stimulus. You know how background noise in your home becomes unnoticeable? Your nervous system will adapt to repetitive stimuli providing it is painless.

Sensory Receptor Classification

There are three types of sensory receptors: proprioceptors, exteroceptors and interoceptors. Proprioceptors let us know the position and movement of our skeletal muscles and our joints. Exteroceptors let us know information about our external environment and interoceptors keep close watch on our visceral organs and what they are doing. We can even break these down further. Nociceptors pick up on pain, thermoreceptors pick up on temperature, mechanoreceptors pick up on physical distortion and chemoreceptors pick up on chemical concentrations.

Nociceptors are very common in the skin. They are also found internally in bones, blood vessels and joints. These receptors have large fields of reception. Fibers called Type A fibers carry sensations of fast pain. This would be like the pain caused from a deep cut. Type C fibers carry slow pain which is more of an aching pain.

Thermoreceptors are located in the dermis, muscles, hypothalamus and liver. We actually have more cold receptors than hot receptors. These receptors are very active when temperature changes, but they adapt quickly and help you to become comfortable.

Mechanoreceptors pick up on any distortion of plasma membranes. If our membranes are stretched, twisted or contorted in any way, the mechanoreceptors will pick up on it. There are also three types of mechanoreceptors. The tactile receptors pick up on touch and vibration, baroreceptors pick up on pressure changes in walls of vessels and parts of the digestive and respiratory tract and proprioceptors will closely monitor position of joints and skeletal muscles.

Tactile receptors come in two forms: fine touch and pressure receptors and crude touch and pressure receptors. The difference is obvious in the names themselves! Fine touch receptors give us detailed information about the stimulation. We can tell the location, size, texture and movement of the stimulating object. The crude touch and pressure receptors don't give us as specific a localization as the fine touch receptors. They are a lot less precise. There are six types of tactile receptors in skin alone: free nerve endings, root hair plexus, tactile corpuscles, lamellated corpuscles, tactile discs and ruffini corpuscles.

Sensory neurons that deliver sensation to the CNS are called first order neurons. The axon of that sensory neuron forms a synapse with an interneuron called the second order neuron which is usually located in the brain stem or spinal cord. If we are to become aware of the sensation the second order neuron will form a synapse on a third order neuron in the thalamus. The third order neuron will then form a synapse with a neuron of the sensory cortex of the cerebral hemisphere. This allows the right cerebral hemisphere to receive sensory info from the left side of the body and vice versa.

6 Tactile Receptors in Skin

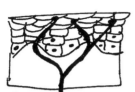

Free Nerve Ending
- sensitive to touch and pressure.

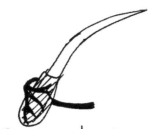

Root hair plexus
- monitor movement across body surface

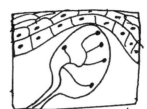

Tactile Corpuscle
(AKA Meissner's Corpuscle)
- sensation of fine touch and pressure

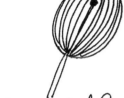

lamellated Corpuscle
(AKA Pacinian Corpuscle)
- sensitive to deep pressure

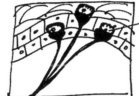

Merkel Cells

Tactile Discs
(AKA Merkel Discs)
- fine touch and pressure receptors with sensitivity to shape and texture.

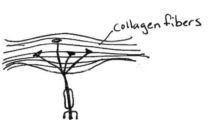

collagen fibers

Ruffini Corpuscles
- sensitive to pressure + distortion of skin but are located in deep dermis

CHAPTER 16

The Autonomic Nervous System

A Flythrough to Complement Your Lab Study

NOTE: This chapter is to be read alongside your lab atlas/manual so that you may examine the autonomic system for the lab portion of your course.

The autonomic nervous system or ANS is not under our conscious control. The ANS is constantly monitoring your homeostasis by checking the cardiovascular, digestive, urinary, reproductive, and respiratory systems. The hypothalamus holds the integrative center for autonomic activity. Somatic nervous system or SNS controls skeletal muscle and the autonomic nervous system or ANS controls visceral effectors like the glands, cardiac muscles and smooth muscle. The ANS distributes motor commands to control activities of target organs as a response to external stimuli. The ANS can be divided into the sympathetic and parasympathetic division. These divisions have opposing effects. The sympathetic division triggers what is often referred to as our "fight or flight" response, whereas the parasympathetic division triggers our "rest and digest" response.

The sympathetic division kicks on only during stress, emergency or physical exertion. The parasympathetic kicks on under resting conditions. In other words, sympathetic nervous system allows your body to work at its maximum in a stressful situation. Maybe you are being chased by an ax murderer? I know, EXTREME! What kind of response do you think your body would have to help you to fight or run? Increased heart rate, blood pressure, respiratory rate? YES! In addition, digestive and urinary function reduce temporarily and more blood will flow to your skeletal muscles. Your metabolic rate will rise and you will have more mental alertness.

The parasympathetic division kicks in when you are relaxed. It causes your body to relax and to spend its efforts on rest and digestion. Your metabolic rate will decrease, your heart rate and blood pressure will decrease, digestive juices will increase, more blood flow to the digestive and urinary tracts which will stimulate urination and defecation.

CHAPTER 17

The Special Senses

A Flythrough to Complement Your Lab Study

NOTE: This chapter is to be read alongside your lab atlas/manual so that you may examine the special senses for the lab portion of your course.

The special senses include olfaction (smell), vision, equilibrium, gustatory (taste), and hearing. Olfaction or the sense of smell arises at the olfactory organs. These are found in the nasal cavity on either side of the nasal septum (the division in the nose that separates nostrils). They are made of olfactory epithelium, which is where the olfactory receptors and stem cells for regeneration are found along with the lamina propria. The lamina propria is mostly areolar tissue, nerves and blood vessels. There are glands called olfactory glands in this tissue and they produce a secretion that forms a thick mucous. When you inhale you are bringing in air that will have scent molecules in it. The movement of these scent molecules across the olfactory epithelium will stimulate the receptors.

Olfactory receptors have an exposed tip that projects outside of the epithelia. Covering that tip are close to 20 dendrites that reach into the mucous. These guys are the ones that pick up on the dissolved scent molecules called odorants. Once an olfactory receptor picks up on an odorant, the olfactory cortex of the cerebral hemispheres interpret it. The axons of the neurons that leave the olfactory epithelium stretch into the brain to reach the olfactory bulbs in the cerebrum. After a scent has been present for some time the olfactory cortex can adapt to it making the scent not as noticeable. Olfactory receptors undergo lots of turnover over time. As we age our receptors are less sensitive and it takes more odorants to stimulate them.

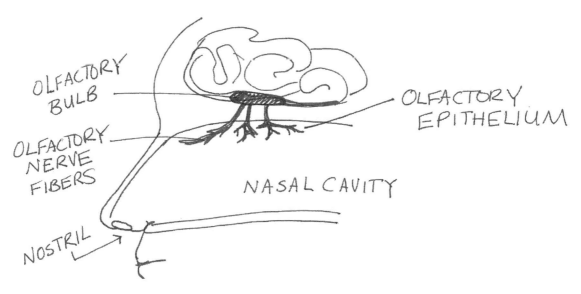

<u>Gustation</u>

Gustation is fancy for taste. <u>Taste receptors</u> are found all over the tongue and also in the pharynx and larynx. The epithelial cells and taste receptors together form structures called <u>taste buds</u>. Human adults have over 10,000. The tongue is covered with <u>lingual papillae</u> of which there are four types: <u>1) foliate papillae, 2) filiform papillae, 3) fungiform papillae and vallate papillae.</u>

The foliate papillae form folds found on the side of the back of the tongue. The filiform papillae help provide friction to move things around in the mouth. The fungiform papillae contain about 5 taste buds each. The vallate papillae can contain as many as 100 taste buds each. All of the taste buds contain receptors and dividing cells called basal cells. Each receptor cell has <u>taste hairs</u> on it that protrude through a narrow opening called the <u>taste pore</u>. These receptors only survive for about 10 days. Taste buds are controlled by cranial nerves. (See text for diagrams showing taste nerves and tract into brain)

There are four primary taste sensations:

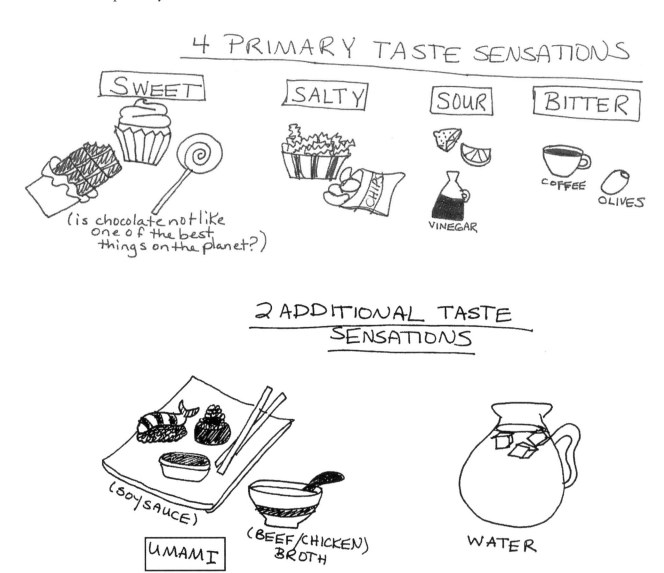

4 PRIMARY TASTE SENSATIONS

SWEET

(is chocolate not like one of the best things on the planet?)

SALTY

CHIPS

SOUR

VINEGAR

BITTER

COFFEE

OLIVES

2 ADDITIONAL TASTE SENSATIONS

(SOY SAUCE)

UMAMI

(BEEF/CHICKEN) BROTH

WATER

BASIC ANATOMY OF THE EYE

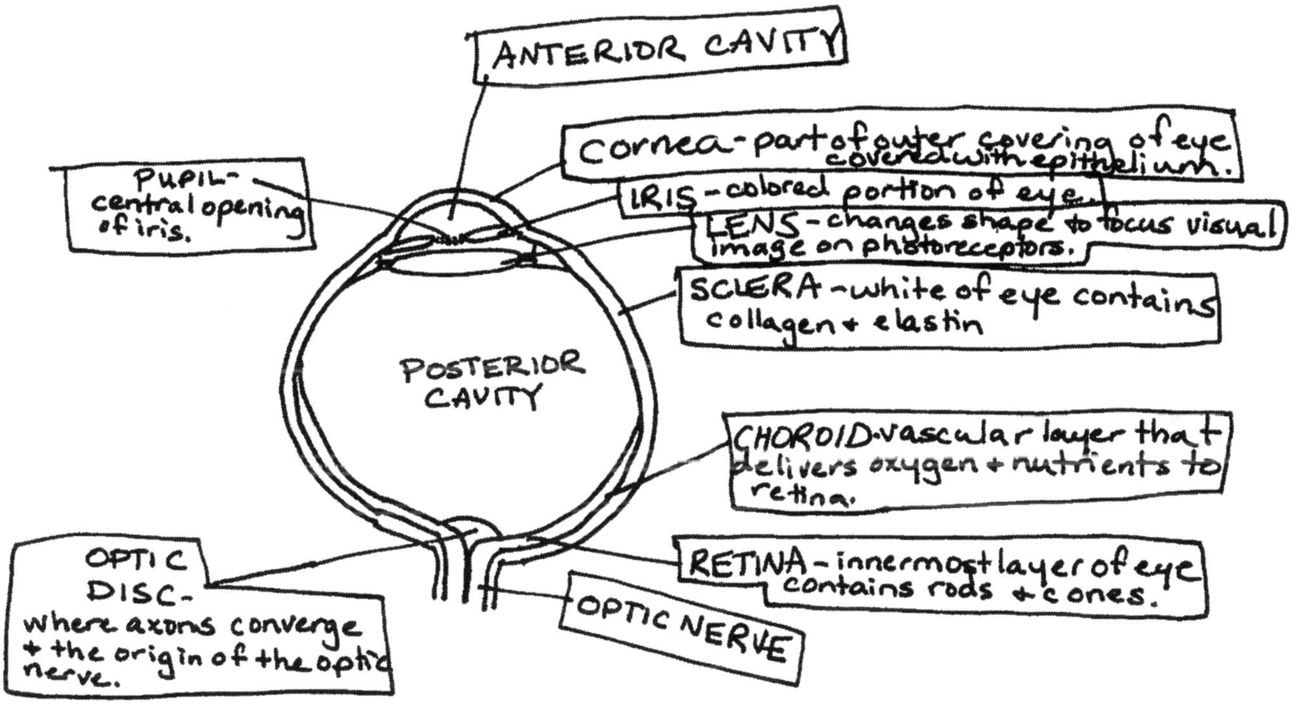

ANTERIOR CAVITY

Cornea - part of outer covering of eye covered with epithelium.

IRIS - colored portion of eye.

LENS - changes shape to focus visual image on photoreceptors.

SCLERA - white of eye contains collagen + elastin

PUPIL - central opening of iris.

POSTERIOR CAVITY

CHOROID - vascular layer that delivers oxygen + nutrients to retina.

RETINA - innermost layer of eye contains rods + cones.

OPTIC DISC - where axons converge + the origin of the optic nerve.

OPTIC NERVE

RODS AND CONES

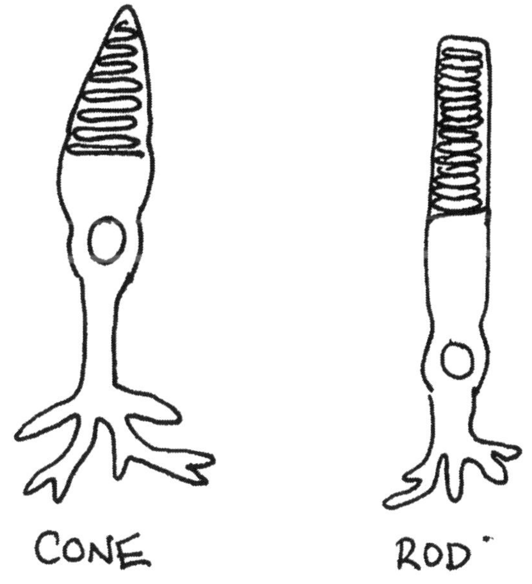

CONE

ROD

Now that you have examined the main parts of the eye let's talk about how it works. The <u>rods</u> and <u>cones</u> of the retina are called <u>photoreceptors</u> because they detect packets of light called <u>photons</u>. Rods do not discriminate against colors of light. They allow us to see in darkness. Cones give us our color vision. We have three types of cones that each contain a different pigment: red, blue or green. Rods tell the CNS if photons are present. Cones will tell us if there is color. Rods and cones both have visual pigment that is located in the outer part of the rod or cone in what are called <u>discs</u>. The rods or cones must first carry out the process of <u>photoreception</u> or detection of light. The visual pigments are derived from <u>rhodopsin</u> or visual purple which is located in the rods. Rhodopsin is made of a protein <u>opsin</u> which is bound to a derivative of vitamin A called <u>retinal</u>. The three color cones contain a different form of opsin and will pick up on a different range of wavelengths of light which will be the basis for color vision.

The visual pathways begin at the photoreceptors and will end at the <u>visual cortex</u> located in the cerebral hemispheres. The visual pathway moves from the photoreceptors to the <u>optic disc</u>, down the optic nerve toward the diencephalon. The two optic nerves converge at the <u>optic chiasm</u> in the diencephalon. Half of the fibers from the optic chiasm head towards the <u>lateral geniculate nucleus</u> on one side of the brain and the other fibers head to the lateral geniculate nucleus on the opposite side of the brain. Visual info then travels to the <u>occipital cortex</u> of the cerebral hemisphere on each side.

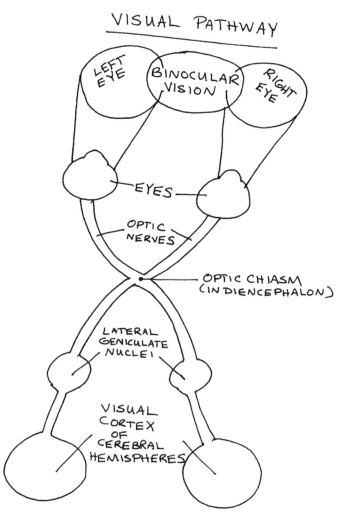

Hearing

The process of hearing can be broken down into 6 steps. <u>Step 1</u>: the sound waves make it to the <u>tympanic membrane</u> through the <u>external acoustic meatus</u>. <u>Step 2</u>: the tympanic membrane begins to move which causes the <u>auditory ossicles</u> to move. This will amplify the sound. <u>Step 3</u>: The <u>stapes</u> creates pressure waves that move through the <u>perilymph</u> of the <u>cochlea</u>. <u>Step 4:</u> The pressure waves will distort the <u>basilar membrane</u> of the cochlea. <u>Step 5</u>: vibration of the basilar membrane will cause <u>hair cells</u> to vibrate. <u>Step 6</u>: Information about the location and intensity of the sound is relayed to the CNS over the <u>cochlear branch</u> of the cranial nerve.

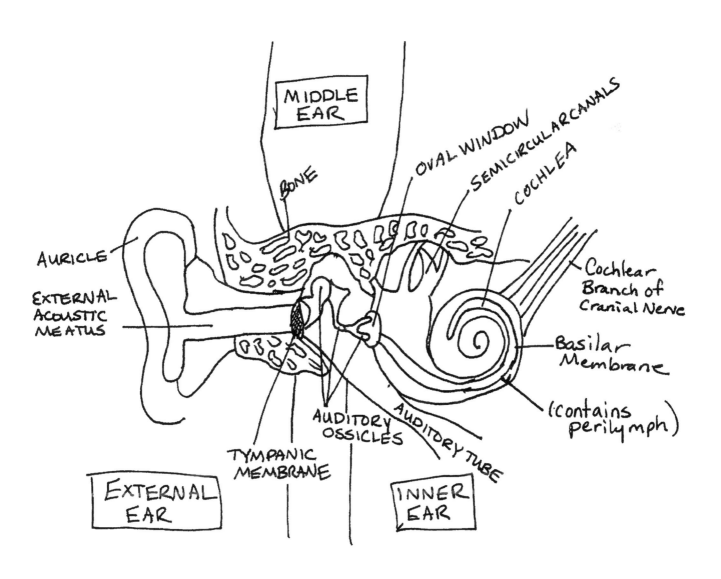

CHAPTER 18

The Endocrine System

The human body uses chemical messengers to communicate. There are about 30 chemical messengers called <u>hormones</u> that the body uses in this communication process. These chemical messengers are regulatory. They help to regulate your sleep, mood, hunger, body temperature and metabolism. The hormones do this along with the help of the nervous system.

To keep our bodies in homeostasis, our cells must be coordinated throughout the body. Neurons control cells or groups of cells throughout the body. Not all cells are directly innervated by the nervous system. The nervous system handles crisis management in a very short-term way. Not all of the body's processes are short-term processes—like growing for example! That's where the endocrine system comes in. It will manage long-term changes in the body. It will use chemical messengers to relay info between cells. Do you remember gap junctions? Cells can communicate through them by passing ions and molecules back and forth through these gaps. This is called <u>direct communication</u>. It is considered direct when the cells are the same type and in close contact with one another. You will find this kind of close communicating relationship in cardiac muscle cells. You definitely want all the cells on the same page, contracting together. It is super important they act as one entity. The majority of communication between cells occurs by the release and acceptance of chemical messages. This is how cells talk to one another. One cell may release a chemical into the extracellular fluid surrounding other cells. This tells the other cells what their neighbors are doing. This helps the tissue containing these cells to coordinate their activities at the local level. This coordination of cells within a single tissue is called <u>paracrine communication</u>. Some examples of these paracrine chemicals or factors are the <u>growth factors</u>. When a chemical messenger is released in one tissue and is transported in the blood stream to alter the activities of other cells in different tissues, we call this a hormone. Most cells release paracrine factors but specialized ones produce hormones.

Every hormone has <u>target cells</u>. These are cells that have the very specific receptors needed to bind and read the hormone when it arrives. This makes a lot of sense! Think about how at any given time you have multiple hormones coursing through your blood. How can we be sure the right hormones affect the right parts of the body? We don't need thyroid hormone binding to the ovaries! Since hormones can only bind with their target cells, this ensures that the right hormones bind in the right places and those places ONLY! Make sense? The hormones fit with the receptors in their target cells like a lock and key or two puzzle pieces. This means a hormone that doesn't belong won't be able to fit in that receptor on that particular target cell. Awesome!

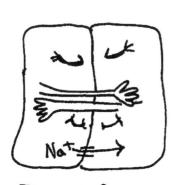

Direct Communication

(must be in direct contact, share info thru gap junctions)

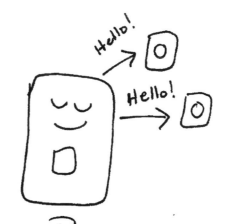

Paracrine Communication

Communication thru extracellular fluid to nearby cells

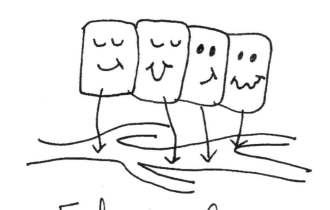

Endocrine Communication

Puts hormones into bloodstream where messages will travel to other parts of body.

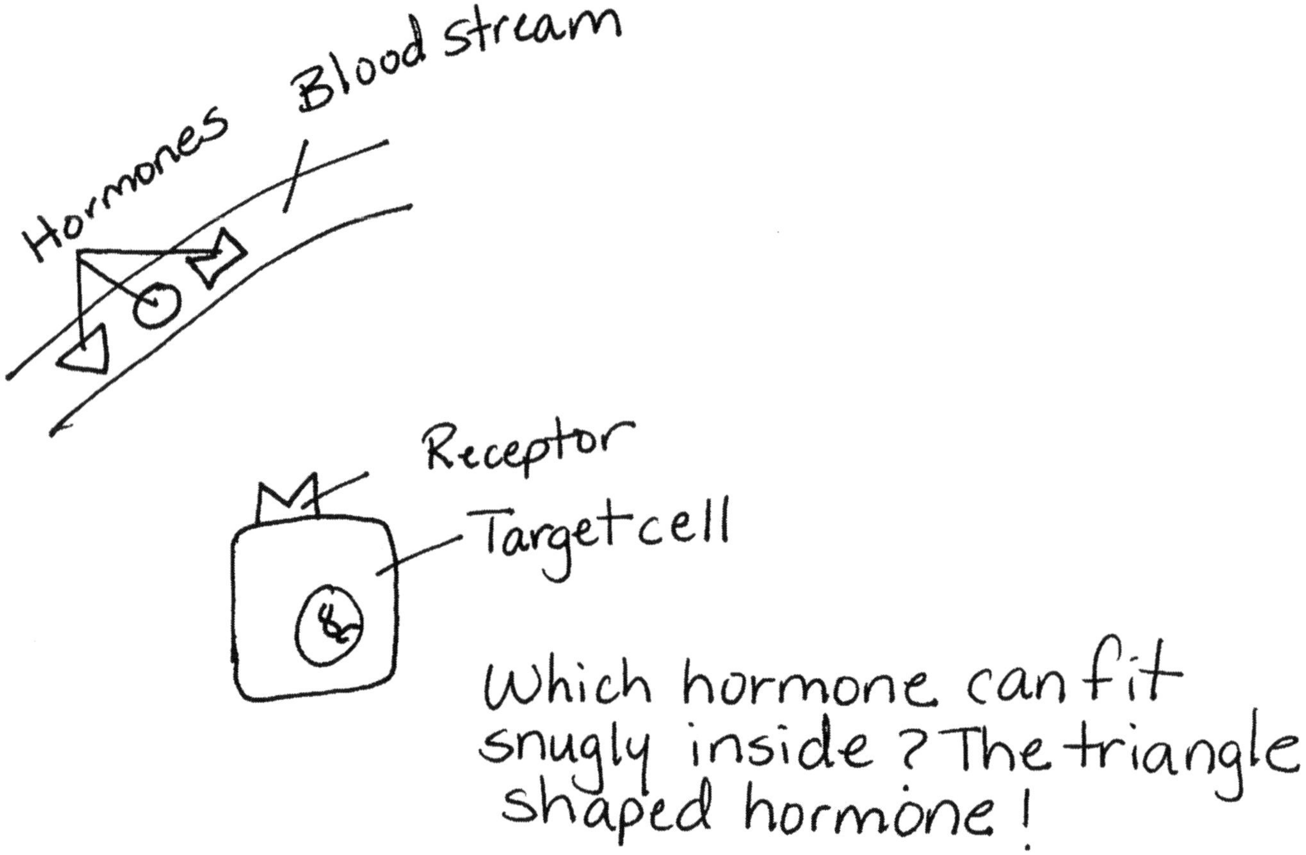

Hormones Blood stream

Receptor
Target cell

Which hormone can fit snugly inside? The triangle shaped hormone!

So once they get to their target cells how do they work? Hormones work by changing the activities of target cells by changing the types, amounts or activities of enzymes and proteins. It could cause an enzyme or protein to be formed by the process of transcription and translation or even turn an existing enzyme or membrane channel on or off. By doing this, a hormone can easily change the structure or chemical properties of the target cell. Since there are lots of target cells for each hormone and since they can be anywhere in the body, one hormone can change the metabolism of multiple tissues or organs at the same time. Wow! Hormones make changes for much longer periods of time. It could be hours, days and sometimes even long coordinated maintenance of processes over a lifetime. That being said hormones are not very good at responding to short term crisis management. The nervous system handles our short term changes.

We can divide hormones into 3 classes on the basis of their chemical structure:

3 Classes of Hormones

Amino Acid Derivatives
- very small
- made from amino acids tyrosine and tryptophan

Tyrosine Based ex.
- Thyroid Hormones

- Epinephrine ⎤
- Norepinephrine ⎬ called Catecholamines as a group
- Dopamine ⎦

Tryptophan Based ex.
- Melatonin

Peptide Hormones
- made of chains of amino acids
- made from glycoproteins and short polypeptides or small proteins.

Glycoprotein Based ex.
- Thyroid Stimulating Hormone ⎫
- Luteinizing Hormone ⎬
- Follicle Stimulating Hormone ⎭

Short Polypeptide or Small Protein Based ex.
- Antidiuretic Hormone
- Oxytocin
- Insulin
- Growth Hormone
- Prolactin

Lipid Derivatives
- two classes: eicosanoids, derived from arachidonic acid and steroid hormones derived from cholesterol.

Eicosanoids ex.
- leukotrienes
- Prostaglandins

Steroid Hormones ex.
- androgen
- estrogen
- progesterone
- corticosteroids
- calcitriol

Secretion of Hormones

Hormones are released where there is a direct link to the blood supply so that the hormones can quickly enter the bloodstream to set out to find their target cells. Hormones can travel in the blood freely (on their own) or bound to a transport protein. Hormones that move freely only remain functional for less than one hour. Once a hormone binds to a target cell it will be absorbed and broken down by cells of the liver or kidneys, or may even be broken down by enzymes in the blood or tissue fluids. Thyroid and steroid hormones last in circulation for much longer because most of them attach to a transport protein. An equilibrium state exists between the bound and free forms of these hormones. As the free ones are inactivated the bound ones are released to replace them. At any time the bloodstream will have a reserve of bound hormones.

Hormone Action

When hormones bind to their target cell's receptors this will cause the activity of the cells to change. It may promote a change in membrane permeability, the activation or inactivation of enzymes, or change in genetic activity. For a hormone to affect a target cell it must interact with its receptor. These receptors can be found on the target cell's membrane or within the target cell. The receptors for catecholamines, peptide hormones and eicosanoids are in the plasma membranes of their target cells. The catecholamines and peptide hormones are not lipid soluble so they cannot pass through the lipid bilayer of the plasma membrane. They must bind extracellularly. Eicosanoids are lipid soluble so they can pass across the plasma membrane and will bind to receptors on the inner surface of the plasma membrane. Communication between the hormone and the target cell uses first and second messengers. The first messenger is the hormone that binds to the membrane on the outside. A second messenger is a helper molecule that appears due to the meeting of the first messenger and receptor. Important second messengers are: cyclic AMP (cAMP) which is a derivative of ATP, cyclic GTP (cGTP) which is a derivative of GTP, and calcium (Ca2+). The link between the first and second messenger is called a G protein. A G protein is an enzyme complex attached to a membrane receptor. G proteins become active when a hormone binds to its receptor at the membrane surface.

G proteins and cAMP

When the G protein is activated it activates the enzyme adenylate cyclase which will convert ATP to cAMP. cAMP then will act as a second messenger by activating a kinase which will attach a high energy phosphate group to another molecule by the process known as phosphorylation. This could open ion channels in the cell for example. The cytoplasm contains another enzyme called phosphodiesterase (PDE) which inactivates cAMP by converting it to AMP.

G proteins and Ca2+

An activated G protein can start the opening of calcium ion channels in the plasma membrane or cause the release of calcium ions from intracellular compartments. The G protein will activate the enzyme phospholipase C (PLC) which triggers a receptor cascade beginning with diacylglycerol

(DAG) and <u>inositol triphosphate</u> (IP3) from the membrane's phospholipids. IP3 diffuses into cytoplasm and starts the release of Ca2+ from reserves in the cell. The combo of DAG and the intracellular calcium ions activates <u>protein kinase C</u> (PKC) which will lead to phosphorylation of calcium channel proteins. This will cause the channels to open and allows Ca2+ to enter the cell. Positive feedback will click on and more Ca2+ will flow in. The calcium acts as a messenger along with an intracellular protein called <u>calmodulin</u>. Calmodulin binds Ca2+ and then activates certain enzymes in the cytoplasm. Calmodulin activation is involved in the stimulatory effects that follow epinephrine or norepinephrine release (we'll talk about those soon).

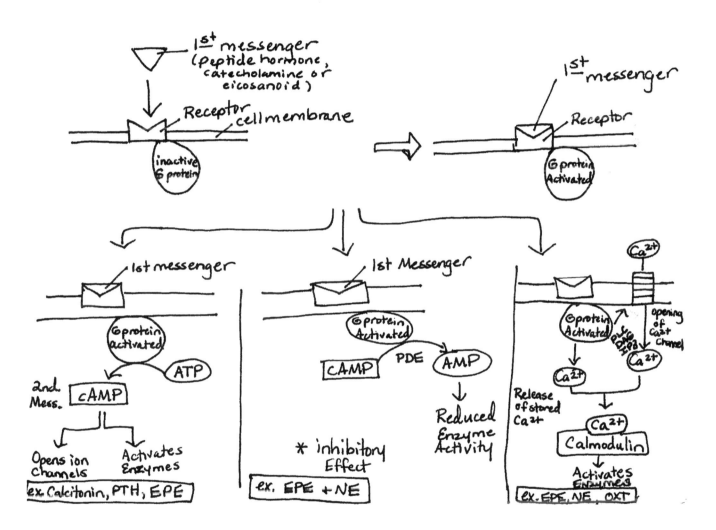

<u>Hormones That Bind With Receptors Inside the Cell</u>

Steroid and thyroid hormones can slip right into the cell. There is no need for a G protein or second messenger. These guys bind with receptors in the nucleus or cytoplasm. Following the binding of a steroid hormone to a receptor is the activation/deactivation of specific genes which can alter the rate of DNA transcription in the nucleus. Since we hopefully remember what transcription is, by changing the rate of it, we are therefore also affecting the rate of protein synthesis. By affecting the rate of protein or enzyme synthesis we are also affecting metabolic rate. Thyroid hormones also cross the cell membrane and bind with a receptor in the nucleus and on mitochondria. Just like with steroid hormones, the binding of the hormone to the receptor in the nucleus will change the rate of DNA transcription in the nucleus. The binding of the hormone to the mitochondria will increase ATP production in the cell.

Control of Endocrine Activity

The hypothalamus gives the highest level of endocrine control. It connects the activities of the nervous and endocrine systems. The hypothalamus itself acts as an endocrine organ by producing two hormones. Those two hormones are released at the posterior pituitary. The hypothalamus also exerts direct control over the adrenal glands. The adrenal glands secrete epinephrine and norepinephrine, but only in response to an action potential from the nervous system. The endocrine system sends commands by changing the amount of hormones secreted. For example when blood glucose climbs, the pancreas increases secretion of insulin which will lower blood glucose. As insulin rises glucose levels go down, as the glucose levels move back towards normal, the rate of insulin secretion returns to normal resting levels. That, my friends, is NEGATIVE FEEDBACK!

The Pituitary Gland

The pituitary gland is also known as the hypophysis. It is well protected by the sphenoid bone of the skull. It is right below the hypothalamus. The pituitary gland has anterior and posterior lobes and releases nine peptide hormones. Seven hormones are released from the anterior portion and two from the posterior portion. The anterior pituitary or adenohypophysis has three regions, the pars distalis, pars tuberalis and the pars intermedia. A rich capillary network fills the anterior pituitary gland so that all cells have instant access to the bloodstream. The hypothalamus controls the production of hormones in the anterior pituitary gland by secreting regulatory hormones. There are two classes of regulatory hormones: releasing and inhibiting hormones. Releasing hormones (RH) stimulate the creation and secretion of one or more hormones at the anterior lobe. The inhibiting hormones (IH) prevent the creation and secretion of hormones from the anterior lobe.

Hormones of the Anterior Lobe

The hormones of the anterior lobe are called tropic, meaning "turning on" hormones. They will switch on other endocrine glands or support the work of other organs.

Thyroid Stimulating Hormone or TSH triggers the thyroid gland itself and causes it to secrete thyroid hormones.

Adrenocorticotropic Hormone or ACTH stimulates the release of steroid hormones by the adrenal gland, causing it to produce glucocorticoids which are hormones that affect glucose metabolism.

Gonadotropins regulate the activity of the gonads (testes and ovaries). They stimulate the production of reproductive cells and hormones. There are two gonadotropins: Follicle Stimulating Hormone or FSH and Luteinizing hormone or LH. FSH promotes follicle development in the ovaries and along with LH will stimulate the secretion of estrogen. FSH in males will help with sperm production. LH causes ovulation or the release of an egg. It also, as mentioned before, assists with the release of estrogen. In additional to estrogen, it will help with the secretion of progesterone which helps prepare the uterus for pregnancy. In men LH assists with the production of androgens like testosterone.

Prolactin or PRL is part of a network of hormones that stimulate milk production in the mammary glands.

Growth Hormone or GH stimulates cell growth and division by increasing the rate of protein synthesis. Skeletal muscle cells and chondrocytes are most sensitive to GH, but most all tissues will respond in some fashion.

Melanocyte Stimulating Hormone or MSH stimulates the melanocytes of the skin causing them to release more melanin, a brown/black pigment.

The Posterior Lobe of the Pituitary Gland

The posterior lobe is also called the neurohypophysis because it contains the axons of hypothalamic neurons. These neurons make antidiuretic hormone or ADH and oxytocin or OXT. The posterior lobe serves as an exit point for these hormones. ADH is released when there is a rise in the solute concentration in the blood or a fall in blood volume or pressure. ADH acts on kidneys to retain water and slow down urination. It will also cause vasoconstriction of peripheral blood vessels which help to elevate blood pressure.

Oxytocin OXT in women will cause smooth muscle contraction in the wall of the uterus during labor and delivery. It can also cause milk ejection from the mammary gland. In men OXT stimulates smooth muscle contractions in the ductus deferens or sperm duct and prostate gland which may help in the ejection of sperm.

Thyroid Gland

The thyroid gland hugs the trachea just below the thyroid cartilage. There are two lobes of the thyroid which are linked in the middle by the isthmus. If something goes wrong with the thyroid it typically enlarges. The thyroid has large follicles which are hollow spheres. The follicle cells are around a follicle cavity that contains a syrupy fluid containing lots of proteins. The thyroid is highly vascular so that it can deliver nutrients and regulatory hormones to the thyroid but also to accept the secretory products of the thyroid. The follicle cells make a protein called thyroglobulin which contain the amino acid tyrosine (which is a component of thyroid hormones). Steps required in the formation of thyroid hormones: 1) To make a thyroid hormone iodide ions must be taken in from the diet through the digestive tract. TSH sensitive carrier proteins will transport the iodide ions into the cytoplasm. 2) The iodide will then diffuse to the apical surface of the follicle cell where they lose an electron and will be converted to iodine by the enzyme called thyroid peroxidase. This reaction sequence will attach one or two iodine atoms to the tyrosine part of a thyroglobulin molecule within the cavity of the follicle. 3) Tyrosine molecules with iodine molecules attached will become linked together by covalent bonds forming molecules of thyroid hormones that remain incorporated into the thyroglobulin. The hormone thyroxine or T4 contains four iodine atoms, triiodothyronine or T3 contains three iodine atoms. Each molecule of thyroglobulin contain four to eight molecules of T4 or T3 or both. The control of how much thyroid hormone is released is directly related to the amount of circulating TSH. TSH helps iodide to transport into the follicle cells of the thyroid and stimulates the production of thyroglobulin and thyroid peroxidase. TSH also causes the release of thyroid hormones. When TSH is present, here's what will happen: 4) follicle cells remove thyroglobulin from the follicles by the process of endocytosis, 5) enzymes of lysosomes break down the thyroglobulin, then the amino acids and thyroid hormones enter the cytoplasm. The amino acids are recycled and used to make more thyroglobulin, 6) the released molecules of T3 and T4 diffuse across the membrane and enter the bloodstream. T4 makes up about 90 percent of all thyroid secretions, 7) 75 percent of the T4 and 70 percent of the T3 molecules entering the bloodstream become attached to transport proteins called thyroid-binding globulins or TBGs. Most of the rest of the T4 and T3 in circulation attach to transthyretin, or to albumin, a plasma protein. Only the remaining small quantities of thyroid hormones that are not bound are free to diffuse into peripheral tissues. Equilibrium will exist between the amount of bound and unbound thyroid hormones. The bloodstream normally has a week's worth of thyroid hormones.

Functions of Thyroid Hormones

Thyroid hormones can affect almost every cell in the body. When they enter a target cell they bind to receptors in the cytoplasm and the nucleus as well as on the surface of mitochondria. The thyroid hormones that bind to receptors in the cytoplasm are held in storage. If levels of thyroid hormone decline, the thyroid hormones held in storage will be released into the cytoplasm. The thyroid hormone that binds to mitochondria will increase the rate of ATP production. The binding in the nucleus will activate genes that control the production of enzymes that help make and use energy. They can also activate genes that code for the creation of enzymes involved in glycolysis and ATP production. All of this will increase the metabolic rate of the cell as a whole. This is referred to as the calorigenic effect. The cell will consume more energy and generate more heat.

Iodine

Iodine comes from our diet and each day the follicle cells of the thyroid gland absorb iodine in order to function. We gain a lot of our dietary iodine through table salt.

C Cells

The C or clear cells are found scattered amongst the follicle cells of the thyroid. They produce the hormone calcitonin or CT. CT helps to regulate Ca2+ in body fluids. We mentioned this hormone and its details in chapter 6.

Parathyroid Glands

The parathyroid glands are four little glands found embedded on the back of the thyroid gland. Parathyroid glands secrete <u>parathyroid hormone or PTH</u>. We also mentioned this hormone and its details in chapter 6. The PTH will raise Ca2+ concentrations in body fluids.

Adrenal Glands

The adrenal glands consist of a <u>medulla</u> or center and a <u>cortex</u> or outer covering. There is one atop each kidney. The adrenal cortex is filled with stored lipids and produces more than two dozen steroid hormones which are called <u>corticosteroids</u>. They turn on transcription of certain genes in the nuclei of their target cells and will help determine their transcription rates. This will result in a change in the amount of enzymes in the cytoplasm which can affect metabolism. There are three zones in the adrenal glands. Each zone produces different hormones.

The <u>zona glomerulosa</u> is the outer edge of the adrenal cortex and makes <u>mineralocorticoids</u>. Mineralocorticoids are steroid hormones that will directly affect the electrolyte composition of your body fluids. <u>Aldosterone</u> is the primary mineralocorticoid produced here. Aldosterone will cause the body to conserve sodium ions and rid itself of potassium ions. It will cause the retention of sodium ions by the kidney, sweat glands, and pancreas. It prevents loss of sodium ions in each of the aforementioned organ secretions. While hoarding the sodium ions the same organs are losing potassium ions. The hoarding of sodium ions will cause the kidneys to reabsorb more water as well as the salivary glands and pancreas. Aldosterone also increases the sensitivity of salt receptors on the tongue which causes one to crave more salt.

The <u>zona fasciculata</u> produces steroid hormones know as <u>glucocorticoids</u> because they affect glucose metabolism. When stimulated by ACTH from the anterior pituitary the zona fasciculata secretes <u>cortisol</u> and <u>corticosterone</u>. The liver converts some of the cortisol into <u>cortisone</u>. Glucocorticoids speed up the rate of glucose creation and glycogen formation in the liver. Adipose tissue releases fatty acids into the blood and other tissues begin to break down fatty acids and proteins instead of glucose. Glucocorticoids also have anti-inflammatory effects. They inhibit the activities of white blood cells in the immune system. Glucocorticoids slow the movement of phagocytic cells to an injury site and mast cells exposed to these steroids are less likely to release <u>histamine</u> which causes inflammation.

The <u>zona reticularis</u> under stimulation of ACTH, produces small quantities of androgens which are the sex hormones produced in large quantities in the testes. Once in the bloodstream, some of these androgens are converted to estrogen which is the dominant sex hormone in females. Adrenal androgens in males produce pubic hair before puberty but do not do much in adulthood for men. In adult women they promote muscle mass and blood cell formation as well as support sex drive.

The Adrenal Medulla

The adrenal medulla produces <u>epinephrine</u> and <u>norepinephrine</u>. Sympathetic stimulation dramatically raises the rate of hormone release. Epinephrine or EPE makes up 75-80 percent of the secretions of the adrenal medulla. The rest is norepinephrine or NE. These hormones will speed up the use of cellular energy and activate energy reserves. In skeletal muscles EPE and NE will activate glycogen reserves and speed up the rate of glucose breakdown to provide ATP. This allows muscles to work at maximum capacity. In adipose tissue, the fat is broken down into fatty acids which will enter the bloodstream for other tissues to make ATP. In the liver, glycogen molecules are broken down into glucose molecules, which are released into the blood to be used by neural tissue. In the heart there will be an increase in the rate and force of cardiac muscle contraction—your heart rate will rise!

The Pineal Gland

The pineal gland of the brain creates melatonin from serotonin. In some mammals melatonin slows down the rate of maturity of sperm, eggs and reproductive organs. In other words, it is thought to help play a role in the timing of sexual maturation. Melatonin is also an antioxidant. It is thought to help protect the CNS from free radicals which damage cells. It may also be involved in maintaining basic circadian rhythm. Circadian rhythms are daily changes in your physiological processes that follow regular day and night patterns.

The Pancreas

The pancreas has both endocrine and exocrine functions. We will talk about the exocrine function in the digestive chapter. The endocrine pancreas is made of clusters of endocrine cells called pancreatic islets. The pancreatic islets are surrounded by extra permeable capillaries. Each islet consists of four types of cells. The alpha cells produce the hormone glucagon which will raise the blood glucose levels by increasing the rates of glycogen breakdown and glucose release in the liver. The beta cells produce the hormone insulin which lowers blood glucose by increasing the rate of glucose uptake and use by most body cells and by causing the muscles and liver the synthesize glycogen. Delta cells produce a hormone identical to growth hormone-inhibiting hormone or GH-IH GH-IH suppresses the release of glucagon and insulin, slows the rate of food absorption and slows the rate of enzyme release in the digestive tract. F cells produce the hormone pancreatic polypeptide or PP which inhibits gallbladder contractions and regulates the production of some enzymes of the pancreas. Let's focus in on insulin and glucagon for a bit.

Insulin is a peptide hormone released by beta cells when the blood glucose levels are above normal. Most cells in the body have receptors for insulin—these cells are called insulin-dependent. Insulin will affect target cells by accelerating glucose uptake. Transport proteins will move glucose into the cells. Insulin will also use and increase ATP production. When more glucose enters the cells, more will be used. When extra glucose enters the cells this will also stimulate glycogen formation and storage. Insulin will also stimulate amino acid absorption and protein synthesis to help maintain glucose levels by preventing the conversion of amino acids to glucose. Insulin also stimulates the absorption of fatty acids and glycerol by adipocytes which will store those components as triglycerides. The adipocytes will also absorb more glucose which can be used in the synthesis of more triglycerides.

MAIN POINT: Insulin is secreted when glucose is in excess. It will cause the body to use glucose to support the body's growth and repair and will make and store carbohydrate (glycogen) and lipid (triglyceride) reserves. This all will help to bring glucose levels with the normal range.

Glucagon

When blood glucose levels are below normal range the alpha cells will secrete glucagon. When glucagon binds to the receptor in its target cell it will activate adenylate cyclase. cAMP will then activate enzymes in the cytoplasm. These effects will follow: Glycogen in the skeletal muscle and liver cells will be broken down and metabolized for energy. Triglycerides will be broken down in adipose tissue. The adipocytes will then release fatty acids into the blood stream for tissues to use. Finally, liver cells will produce and release glucose by converting amino acids from the bloodstream into glucose and putting it into circulation.

MAIN POINT: These processes will reduce glucose utilization and cause the release of more glucose into the bloodstream, pushing the levels more towards normal.

NOTE: We will cover hormones released by the kidneys, intestines, heart and gonads in the corresponding chapters.

The extracellular fluids contain a mixture of hormones at any given time which are constantly in flux. Cells must respond to multiple hormones at once. When a cell receives instructions from more than one hormone at once the outcomes can be: Synergistic, meaning the hormones work together so that the result is greater than the effort of an individual hormone. The result can be antagonistic, which means opposing effects. The end result will be a weaker effect than those produced by the individual hormones. One hormone could have a permissive effect, as in it helps or allows another hormone to work. Without it the other hormone could not have an effect. Finally, it could have integrative effects where the hormones produce different but also complementary effects.

CHAPTER 19

Blood and Blood Vessels

Blood is the liquid part of the cardiovascular system. We know that the heart pumps that blood around right? The heart also uses blood vessels to help it accomplish that task. We need blood to circulate around the body because it delivers all of the necessary nutrients and oxygen all of our cells need as well as picks up all of the wastes and carbon dioxide our cells don't need! Another awesome thing that blood does is carry cells that fight infection around the body—that's kind of a big deal!

Do you remember how we learned that blood is a fluid connective tissue? Remember that connective tissues are tissues that have specialized cells and a matrix that the cells are suspended in? The matrix for blood is fluid. Blood is used for transporting dissolved gasses like CO_2 and O_2. It will also transport nutrients, hormones and wastes created by metabolism. Blood will also regulate the pH and ions of interstitial fluid. It will also respond to cuts or breaks in blood vessel walls by causing clotting. Blood transports <u>white blood cells or WBCs</u> to fight infection and will help to keep your body temperature stable. Blood absorbs heat from skeletal muscle tissues and redistributes it to other tissues in the body. What makes up blood?

The matrix of blood is called <u>plasma</u>. The plasma has what are called <u>formed elements</u> in it. Plasma makes up around 46-63% of the volume of whole blood. 92% of plasma is water! The formed elements of blood are <u>platelets, WBCs and red blood cells or RBCs</u>. These account for 37-54% of the volume of whole blood. Blood pH is found between 7.35-7.45. First let's go into detail about the plasma.

<u>Plasma</u>

Plasma is mostly water but also includes proteins and other solutes. The dissolved proteins are mainly albumin, fibrinogen and globulin. <u>Albumin</u> proteins are helpful for transporting fatty acids, thyroid hormones and some steroid hormones. <u>Globulins</u> either are found as antibodies, or aid in transport and will bind with hormones and other small ions. <u>Fibrinogen</u> is going to aid in clotting.

<u>The Formed Elements</u>

<u>Red Blood Cells (RBCs)</u> account for 99.9 percent of the formed elements and contain <u>hemoglobin (Hb)</u> which is responsible for carrying oxygen and carbon dioxide. RBCs are so different! Each one is a disk shape with a concave (dented in) middle.

RBC

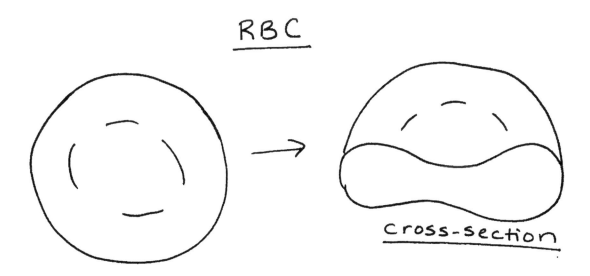

cross-section

This cool shape gives the RBC a large surface area-to-volume ratio. This will allow the oxygen to be absorbed or released quickly as the RBC passes through capillaries of the lungs and tissues. Its shape will also allow it to be more flexible. It can squeeze and flex as it moves through tiny capillaries. The RBCs can also stack on top of each other and still squeeze through small capillaries without forming blocks or jams. What's extra weird is that when RBCs form, they lose most of their organelles, including the nucleus and are left with only the cytoskeleton. Since they don't have organelles and cannot repair themselves, they have a short life span of only about 120 days.

Hemoglobin or Hb makes up more than 95 percent of a RBC's proteins. It is what is primarily responsible for the cell's ability to transport oxygen and carbon dioxide. Hb is a complex quaternary protein. Each Hb contains a single molecule of <u>heme</u> which holds an iron ion. This iron ion can join with an oxygen, forming what is called <u>oxyhemoglobin</u>. Blood that has oxyhemoglobin is bright red. When there is no oxygen bound with the iron on a hemoglobin this is called <u>deoxyhemoglobin</u> which is a darker red. Each RBC contains around 280 million Hb molecules.

RBCs are broken down and recycled often due to their short life spans. Even the parts of the RBC are broken down. The Hb is broken down into its amino acid components which will be metabolized or released into the bloodstream. The heme unit's iron is taken away and the heme is then called <u>biliverdin</u> (which is greenish). You know how bruises can look greenish? Yep! That's the culprit! Biliverdin converts to <u>bilirubin</u> (orangy-yellow pigment) and then is released into the bloodstream where it sticks to albumin and moves towards the liver to be excreted in bile. In the large intestine, bacteria convert bilirubin to <u>urobilinogen</u> (some of which is released in urine) and <u>stercobilinogen</u>.

How are RBCs made? In adults, <u>red bone marrow</u> is where RBCs and <u>white blood cells or WBCs</u> are produced. The process of making RBCs is called <u>erythropoiesis</u>. This only happens in bones like some vertebrae, sternum, skull, pelvis, ribs, scapulae, femur and humerus.

RBC Maturation

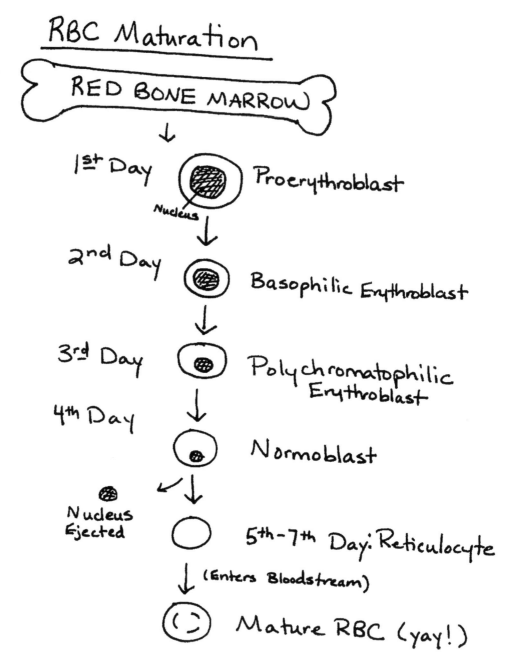

RED BONE MARROW

↓

1st Day — Proerythroblast
Nucleus

2nd Day — Basophilic Erythroblast

3rd Day — Polychromatophilic Erythroblast

4th Day — Normoblast

Nucleus Ejected

5th–7th Day: Reticulocyte

(Enters Bloodstream)

Mature RBC (yay!)

Note: Reticulocytes contain 80% of the Hb of a mature RBC.

White Blood Cells (WBCs)

WBCs look totally different. They do have nuclei and other organelles. WBCs are also known as leukocytes. They are so majorly important because they are our body defenders! They protect us from pathogens, toxins and damaged cells. There are two main categories of WBCs.

WBCs

Agranular leukocytes
- monocytes
- lymphocytes

Granular leukocytes
- neutrophils
- eosinophils
- basophils

WBCs are awesome because they can move throughout the body and don't have to remain only in the blood like the RBCs. WBCs know where infections or damage are because they follow chemical trails (like following bread crumbs) that the damaged tissue puts out. WBCs have the ability to leave the bloodstream by squeezing through the endothelial cells (cells lining the blood vessel) so that they can enter the surrounding tissue. They are all attracted to chemicals that guide them to invaders or damaged tissue—this is called positive chemotaxis. The neutrophils, eosinophils and monocytes can engulf pathogens.

WBCs

Agranular leukocytes
- monocytes
- lymphocytes

Granular leukocytes
- neutrophils
- eosinophils
- basophils

Quick Facts

* Neutrophils, eosinophils, basophils + monocytes are part of the body's <u>non</u>-specific defenses. Stimuli have to activate these defenses. They will respond to any type of threat.

* Lymphocytes are responsible for <u>specific defenses</u>. They respond to specific proteins that are foreign or pathogens.

Neutrophils
- mobile (fast!)
- attack + digest bacteria

Eosinophils
- enguif antibody marked pathogens
- eject toxic compounds onto large objects that can't be engulfed.

Basophils
- eject histamine (which ↑ blood flow) + heparin (prevents clotting) into interstitial fluid.

Monocytes
- acts as a macrophage (aggressive phagocyte)
- Draw fibroblasts in to produce scar tissue.

Lymphocytes
- T cells - defend against invading foreign cells.
- B cells - involved in production of antibodies. Antibodies move through blood, lymph + interstitial fluid.
- Natural Killer Cells - Kill abnormal cells (prevents cancer.)

Platelets

Platelets are in charge of clotting. Platelets will release enzymes and other chemicals to help control the clotting process. They will help to downsize the size of a break in the blood vessel wall by contracting and shrinking themselves. They will also form a temporary patch in the wall of a damaged blood vessel by clumping themselves up.

Blood Vessels

Arteries carry blood away from the heart. When they enter peripheral tissues they become more and more finely branched until they become arterioles. From the arterioles blood would then move into capillaries where diffusion of gases takes place. Once we leave the capillaries, blood would enter small venules which will join to become larger veins that return blood to the heart. All chemical and gas exchange between blood and interstitial fluid takes place across capillary walls.

Vessel Walls

The walls of arteries and veins have three layers, the tunica intima, tunica media and tunica externa. The tunica intima is the inner layer of a blood vessel. It includes endothelial lining and connective tissue with elastic fibers. In an artery—which needs to be tougher, the outer edge of the tunica intima contains a thick layer of elastic fibers called the internal elastic membrane.

The tunica media is the middle layer of a blood vessel. It contains sheets of smooth muscle tissue. This layer is usually the thickest in a small artery. It is separated from the tunica externa by a thin band of elastic fibers called the external elastic membrane. When the smooth muscle contracts, this causes the diameter of the vessel to shrink down. When the smooth muscle relaxes, this causes the diameter of the vessel to open up or dilate.

The tunica externa is the outermost covering of a vessel. This layer has lots of stretchy collagen and elastic fibers. This is going to make the vessel walls strong! Diffusion does not take place through artery and vein walls because the layers are too thick.

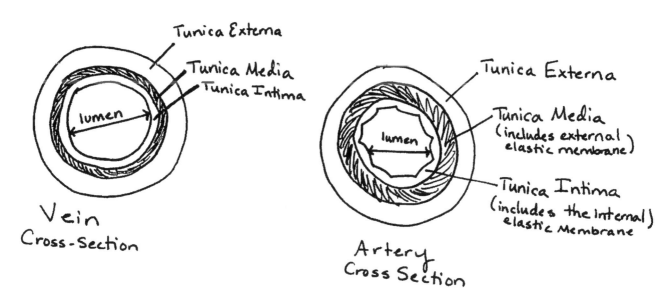

Arteries and Veins

The tunica media of an artery contains lots more smooth muscle and elastic fibers than does a tunica media of a vein. This will help the artery to handle arterial pressure from the heart as it pumps blood into the pulmonary trunk and aorta (chapter 20). Veins usually have valves to help prevent backflow of blood. Arteries are VERY stretchy. When the muscle wall of an artery contracts, this constricts or tightens the artery—this is called vasoconstriction. When the muscle wall of an artery relaxes, this will increase the diameter of the vessel—this is called vasodilation.

Arteries can be classified into elastic, muscular or arterioles. Let's examine elastic first…Elastic arteries carry large amounts of blood away from the heart—these are the big boys! (ex. Pulmonary trunk and aorta) As the name implies these guys are VERY elastic. They can go with the flow and stretch and tolerate the pressure the heart and blood flow put on them. The muscular arteries are smaller or medium sized. These guys are primarily delivering blood to the organs and muscles. They have a thick tunica media that contains lots of smooth muscle cells. The arterioles are much smaller than muscular arteries—these are the lil' guys! Capillaries are teeny tiny—these vessels are interwoven in active tissues. Capillaries are so thin that they allow exchange between the blood and the surrounding interstitial fluids. A capillary is made of an endothelial tube inside a thin basement membrane—no tunica media or tunica externa at all. There are two types of capillaries: continuous capillaries and fenestrated capillaries. Continuous capillaries are found in all tissues except for epithelia and cartilage. In continuous capillaries, the endothelium is a complete smooth lining. This is where water, lipid-soluble materials and small solutes can diffuse into the interstitial fluid. Fenestrated capillaries have pores that allow for rapid passing or exchange of water and solutes between blood and interstitial fluid. These are found in parts of the brain, intestinal tract, kidneys and endocrine system. A capillary bed can also be called a capillary plexus. This is a network of capillaries. One arteriole can branch into dozens of capillaries.

Veins take blood from all tissues and organs and return it to the heart. The walls of veins are thinner than those of arteries because the blood pressure in veins is lower than in arteries. Venules are the smallest venous vessels, they take blood from capillaries. They lack a tunica media. Venules feed into medium sized veins. Medium sized veins have a thin tunica media and have very few smooth muscle cells. Large veins like the vena cavae have all three layers of tunica.

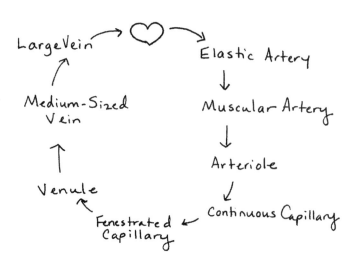

CHAPTER 20

<u>The Heart</u>

Blood flows through a network of blood vessels that stretch between the heart and peripheral tissues. This network of vessels is broken up into two circuits: <u>pulmonary</u> and <u>systemic circuits</u>. The pulmonary circuit carries blood to and from the lungs whereas the systemic circuit carries blood to and from the rest of the body.

REVIEW: -Arteries carry blood away from the heart. (Artery starts with 'A', away starts with 'A')

-Veins carry blood to the heart.

-Capillaries permit exchange of gases, nutrients and wastes.

First we will examine the main parts of the heart (though you can examine your text for detailed anatomical illustrations), then we will talk about how the heart works.

<u>Heart</u>

The human heart has 4 chambers: the <u>right and left atrium</u> and the <u>right and left ventricle</u>. The right side of the heart deals with deoxygenated blood whereas the left deals with oxygenated blood. The heart is right behind the sternum or breastplate and is about the size of a fist. The pointed tip of the heart is called the <u>apex</u>. The heart is positioned in what is called a <u>pericardial sac</u>. The pericardial sac is made of a network of collagen. The heart fits into the pericardial sac like a fist would fit into a squishy partially deflated balloon. The sac is lined by a serous membrane called the <u>parietal pericardium</u>. The <u>visceral pericardium</u> (or epicardium) covers and sticks to the outer surface of the heart. The space between the parietal and visceral pericardium is filled with a fluid called <u>pericardial fluid</u>. This fluid is made by the two previously mentioned membranes. It serves to lubricate and reduce friction between the heart and the pericardial sac with every heartbeat. Can you imagine if you could feel each heartbeat? YUCK!

Heart Basics

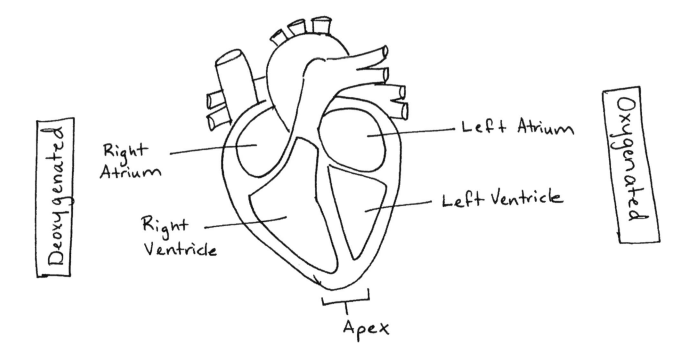

Deoxygenated

Oxygenated

Right Atrium

Left Atrium

Right Ventricle

Left Ventricle

Apex

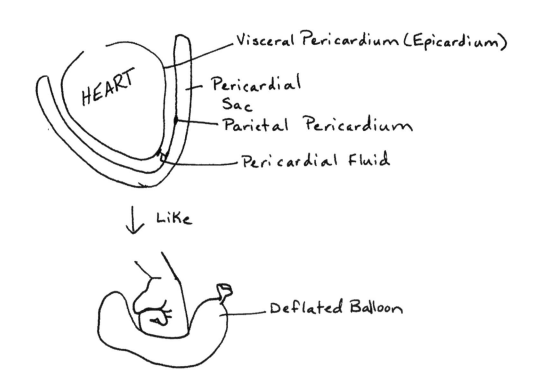

HEART

Visceral Pericardium (Epicardium)

Pericardial Sac

Parietal Pericardium

Pericardial Fluid

↓ Like

Deflated Balloon

Heart Anatomy Basics and Blood Flow Through the Heart

The two atria have thin muscular walls in comparison to the ventricles. The atria are very expandable due to the atrial auricles. The auricle is an expandable extension of the atria, when filled with blood it balloons out a bit, when empty of blood it collapses like a wrinkly ear. The heart wall is made of three layers of tissue: the endocardium, myocardium and epicardium or visceral pericardium. The endocardium lines the inner surface of the heart. It is made of simple squamous epithelium. The myocardium is the muscular wall of the heart—made of cardiac muscle tissue. The epicardium is the previously mentioned serous membrane called the visceral pericardium.

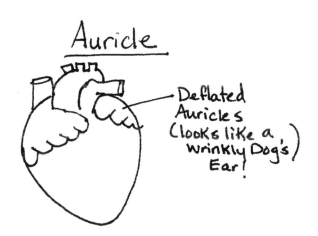

The myocardium is made of cardiac muscle cells that are connected by intercalated discs. In an intercalated disc, the membranes of neighboring cells are connected by desmosomes and gap junctions. Remember those? This way the cells can communicate and share the contraction force from cell to cell and carry on action potentials to make the heart beat or contract. Unlike in skeletal muscle, the cardiac muscle tissue must work together and not in groups. Communication is key! The intercalated discs allow for this connection to occur.

The atria are separated by the <u>interatrial septum</u> and the ventricles are separated by the <u>interventricular septum</u>. The septa are muscular partitions or dividers. The <u>atrioventricular or AV valves</u> include the <u>tricuspid valve</u> and the <u>mitral or bicuspid</u> valve. They permit blood flow in only one direction—from the atria to the ventricles. The right atrium will receive blood from the systemic circuit through the <u>superior and inferior vena cavae</u>. The superior vena cava brings deoxygenated blood back from the head, neck and upper limbs, and the inferior vena cava brings deoxygenated blood back from the trunk and lower limbs. The cardiac veins (see your text to see the anatomy of the coronary vessels) drain the myocardium of deoxygenated blood and return it to the coronary sinus which opens into the right atrium. This will fill the right atrium with deoxygenated blood. During embryonic development up until birth there is an oval shaped opening in the right atrial wall called the <u>foramen ovale</u>. This opening is in the interatrial septum and allows the two atria to be connected in the fetal heart. Why? This will allow blood to flow from the right atria to the left atria while the lungs develop. When the baby is born, the foramen ovale will close and a small oval depression where it once was will be visable, this is called the <u>fossa ovalis</u>. Blood will then travel from the right atrium through the tricuspid valve into the right ventricle. It's easy to remember which valve this one is because it has three cusps or flaps (tri- (three)-cuspid). The cusps of the valves are held down by fibers called the <u>chordae tendineae</u> or tendinous cords. These cords are attached to <u>papillary muscles</u> which are nipple shaped. The AV valves prevent the backflow of blood from the ventricles to the atria when the ventricles are contracting.

*when the ventricles are relaxed, the chordae tendineae are loose, blood flows through the open AV valves from the atria to the ventricles.

*when the ventricles are contracted, blood moving back towards the atria swings the cusps of the valves together, closing the valves. The contraction of the papillary muscles tenses the chordae tendineae, stopping the cusps before they swing backwards into the atria.

The internal surface of the ventricles contain muscular ridges called <u>trabeculae carneae.</u> The <u>semi-lunar valves</u> are the <u>pulmonary and aortic valves</u>. Blood flowing from the right ventricle flows through the pulmonary valve, into the pulmonary trunk, through the <u>left and right pulmonary arteries</u> and into the pulmonary circuit to become oxygenated. Once oxygenated the blood returns to the heart through the left and right pulmonary veins and flows into the left atrium. Blood then moves through the bicuspid or mitral valve which has two cusps (bi-(two)-cuspid) into the left ventricle. The left ventricle is much larger than the right ventricle due to its thick muscular walls. The left ventricle has to push blood through the entire body—through the systemic circuit—that's a huge job. Compare that to the right ventricle that pumps blood to the lungs or pulmonary circuit which is right next door! The left ventricle is six times stronger than the right ventricle. Blood then leaves the left ventricle through the aortic valve and moves into the ascending aorta, aortic arch and finally the descending aorta and out to the body via the systemic circuit.

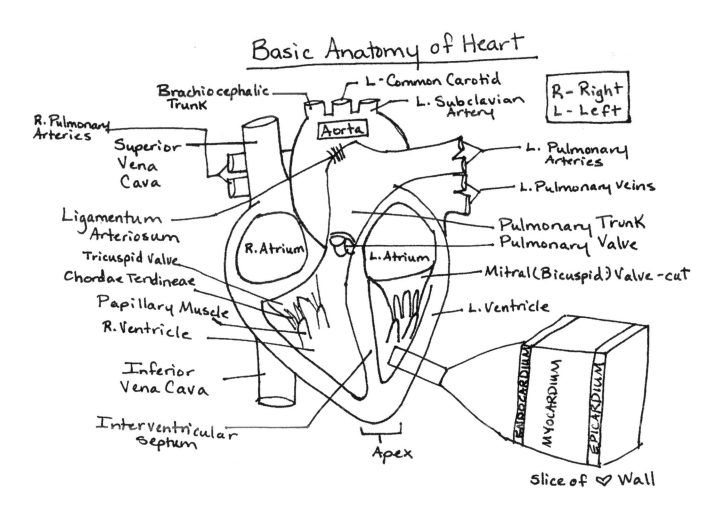

Basic Anatomy of Heart

- 121 -

Blood Flow Through The Heart

Blood returns to heart
via the Superior and
Inferior Vena Cavae

↓

Right Atrium

↓

Tricuspid Valve

↓

Right Ventricle

↓

Pulmonary Valve

↓

Pulmonary Trunk

↓

R + L Pulmonary
Arteries

↓

Lungs (Drops off CO_2 + Picks
up O_2)

↓

Deoxygenated

Blood Returns to heart Via
the L + R Pulmonary
Veins.

↓

Left Atrium

↓

Bicuspid (Mitral) Valve

↓

Left Ventricle

↓

Aortic Valve

↓

Ascending, Arch + Descending
Aorta

↓

Out to body Via Systemic
Circuit

Oxygenated

The heart tissue includes large amounts of collagen and elastic fibers. This gives the heart support and elasticity or stretchiness! It also helps spread the force of contraction and keeps the heart protected from over-expanding.

**please examine your text for the anatomy of the coronary arteries and cardiac veins that make up the blood supply to the heart.

The Conducting System

In a contraction of the heart (heartbeat) the atria contract first and then the ventricles. This makes total sense if you think about it…the atria must contract first so that the blood can move into the ventricles. If the ventricles don't first receive blood then there is no reason for them to contract. To make the heart beat we need the conducting system and the contractile cells. The heartbeat is set by the natural pacemaker called the SA or sinoatrial node. The SA node is part of the conducting system. The conducting system will spread the impulse which will trigger the contractile cells to push blood. When the electrical impulse of the conducting system arrives at the cardiac muscle cell's membrane, it will produce an action potential. Do you remember those from the muscle and nervous system chapters? This action potential or AP will cause the cardiac muscle cell to contract. You don't have to think about your heartbeat do you? It just happens. Aren't you so glad you don't have that responsibility?! Cardiac muscle tissue contracts on its own—this is called automaticity. The conducting system begins with the SA node and is followed by the atrioventricular or AV node. Conducting cells connect the two nodes and will help spread the stimulus throughout the myocardial wall. The impulse then heads through the AV bundle, bundle branches and then the Purkinje fibers which take the stimulus through to the myocardium of the ventricles.

The SA node is found in the wall of the right atrium and has pacemaker cells to help keep the heart rate. Conducting cells will pass the stimulus to contractile cells of both atria so that the action potential can spread across the atrial surfaces by cell to cell contact—remember those intercalated discs? Yeah!

The AV node is in the floor of the right atrium. There will be a slight delay in the impulse here which is great because it will allow the atria to contract before the ventricles. The impulse then is spread along the AV bundle, along the interventricular septum and enters the left and right bundle branches. The impulse then finally moves into the Purkinje fibers.

Conducting System

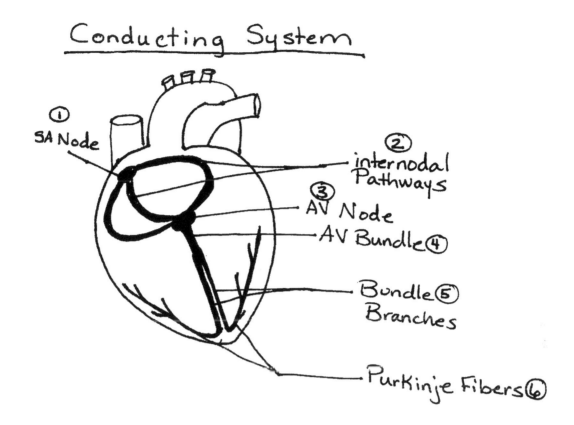

Labels on diagram:
- ① SA Node
- ② Internodal Pathways
- ③ AV Node
- ④ AV Bundle
- ⑤ Bundle Branches
- ⑥ Purkinje Fibers

Contractile Cells

The resting membrane potential of a ventricular contractile cell is -90mV, for an atrial contractile cell it is -80mV. An action potential or AP will happen when a cell's membrane is pushed to threshold which is -75mV. Three things will happen: 1) Once we have reached threshold we will then enter the first phase—rapid depolarization. This is when voltage gated sodium or Na+ channels open and sodium begins to move into the cell rapidly depolarizing the cell membrane or sarcolemma. The cell will depolarize to around +30mV. At this time the sodium channels will close and will stay closed until the membrane potential is at -60mV. At this point the cell will begin pumping sodium out of the cell. Our membrane potential does not go way back down after the sodium channels close because as they are closing the 2) voltage gated calcium or Ca2+ channels are opening and calcium begins entering the cytosol. This positivity coming in in the form of calcium allows the membrane potential to stay near 0mV—this is called the plateau. Calcium channels will begin to slowly close and 3) potassium or K+ channels begin to open. Potassium rushes out of the cell and the cell rapidly repolarizes. This will bring us back to resting membrane potential. After the cell has begun its AP it cannot be stimulated again by normal means, this is called the refractory period. The absolute refractory period is when the membrane cannot respond at all, the relative refractory period is when the membrane can respond to a stronger than normal stimulus.

Do you remember the steps of an AP in a muscle cell? The steps here are very similar. When the AP happens, this produces a contraction in the cardiac muscle cells or a heartbeat. This can happen because the AP will cause an increase in the concentration of calcium around the myofibrils in the cardiac muscle cells. So above we talked about how calcium would come in during the plateau phase, right? This flow of calcium in will also cause the sarcoplasmic reticulum to release more calcium from reserves. In a cardiac muscle cell the AP is longer than that of a skeletal muscle AP. The cell will contract until the plateau phase ends. As the calcium channels close at the end of the plateau phase, the sarcoplasmic reticulum will absorb the remaining calcium or it will be pumped out of the cell causing the cardiac muscle cell to relax.

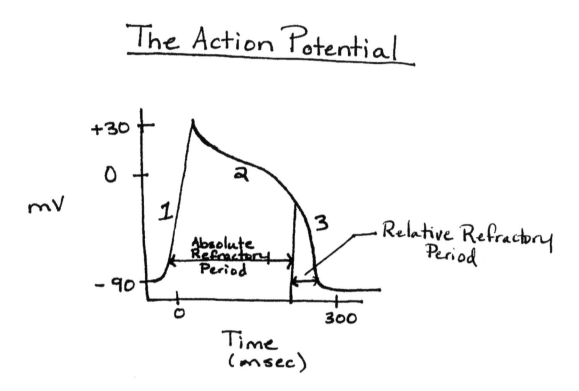

There will be a short rest after each heartbeat which gives the chambers time to relax and get ready for the next of many heartbeats. The period between the start of one heartbeat and the beginning of the next is called a cardiac cycle. During a cardiac cycle each chamber will undergo systole and diastole. Systole is when the chamber contracts and pushes blood, diastole is when the chamber relaxes and fills with blood.

Heart Sounds

Listening to the heart using a stethoscope is called <u>auscultation</u>. There are four heart sounds: <u>S1, S2, S3 and S4</u>. The first sound (or S1) "lubb sound" is caused by the closing of the AV valves (tricuspid and bicuspid). The S2 "dupp" sound is caused by the closing of the semilunar valves (pulmonary and aortic). S3 and S4 are very faint and hard to hear in adults. S3 is the sound of blood flowing into the ventricles and S4 is the sound of atrial contraction.

<u>Cardiac output or CO</u> is defined as the amount of blood pumped by the left ventricle in one minute. This tells us how efficient the ventricles are. You can calculate CO this way:

$$CO = HR \times SV$$

HR=heart rate-beats per minute.

SV=stroke volume-amount of blood pumped out of each ventricle in a single beat.

CHAPTER 21

<u>The Lymphatic System and Immunity</u>

We are in a world filled with pathogens that could thrive inside our bodies. Ew. The lymphatic system is made of the cells, tissues and organs that are in charge of protecting the body from such invaders. It also has the ability to protect us against our own cells that have gone bad, like cancer cells. Do you remember talking about lymphocytes back in the tissue chapter? They will attack pathogens like bacteria or viruses and cancer cells. Our bodies' ability to avoid infection is called <u>immunity</u>. Our bodies have two means of defense: <u>innate defenses</u> and <u>adaptive defenses</u>. Barriers like the skin will keep out or slow down invading pathogens and attack them if they do enter. This is an example of an innate defense—because you were born with it! When bacteria invade a tissue, lymphocytes will launch an attack against that specific bacterium—this is an adaptive defense. The immune system is found in the skin, bones, lymphatic, respiratory, digestive and cardiovascular systems.

The lymphatic system is made of <u>lymph, lymphoid tissues and organs, lymphocytes, phagocytes and lymphatic vessels</u>. Lymph is a clear-ish yellow plasma like fluid. Lymphatic vessels are going to begin in peripheral tissues and connect right into veins. <u>Primary lymphoid tissues and organs</u> are where the lymphocytes are made and where they mature. This would include places like the red bone marrow and the thymus gland. <u>Secondary lymphoid tissues and organs</u> are where lymphocytes become active and are cloned. They are in places like the lymph nodes, muscosa lymphoid tissue (in digestive, respiratory and reproductive tracts) and tonsils.

**Please examine your text for a mapping of the lymphatic vessels and lymph node locations in the body.

The goal in focus for the lymphatic system is to produce and distribute the lymphocytes that will protect us against infection. In order for the lymphocytes to protect us they must be able to get to the areas where there may be an infection or injury. The microphages, macrophages and lymphocytes circulate in the blood and are able to enter or exit the capillaries that are going to most all of the tissues in your body. This gives them access to get to sites of infection or damage. Our capillaries will bring in more fluid to the peripheral tissues than they will take away. This extra fluid will return to the blood stream through the lymphatic vessels mentioned previously. Because there is a continuous loop of extracellular fluid circulating around, this makes it easy to transport lymphocytes, microphages and macrophages from one organ to another. In circulating constantly, this also helps to maintain blood volume. Lymphatic vessels carry lymph from the peripheral tissues to the venous system. The network of lymphatics begins with the tiniest—the <u>lymphatic capillaries</u>. These guys weave through the peripheral tissues. They are wider than capillaries and have thinner walls. They are lined by endothelial cells but the basement membrane is either leaky or not there at all! The endothelial cells are not bound tightly together but they overlap. The area of overlap acts as a one way valve. Fluids and solids, including bacteria and viruses can enter through these leaky valves.

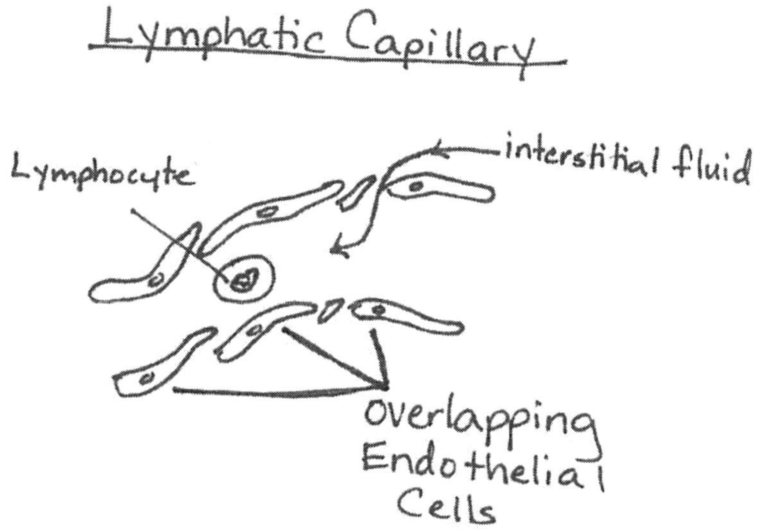

Lymphatic Capillary

Lymphocyte — interstitial fluid

Overlapping Endothelial Cells

From the lymphatic capillaries, lymph will move into the <u>small lymphatic vessels</u> which are a bit larger. These lead towards the trunk of the body. These vessels have walls that are similar to veins and even have valves. These valves make the lymphatic vessels bulge, which give the vessels a beaded appearance. The valves will keep the lymph from back-flowing. When you move, your skeletal muscles will help "push" the lymph towards your thoracic cavity.

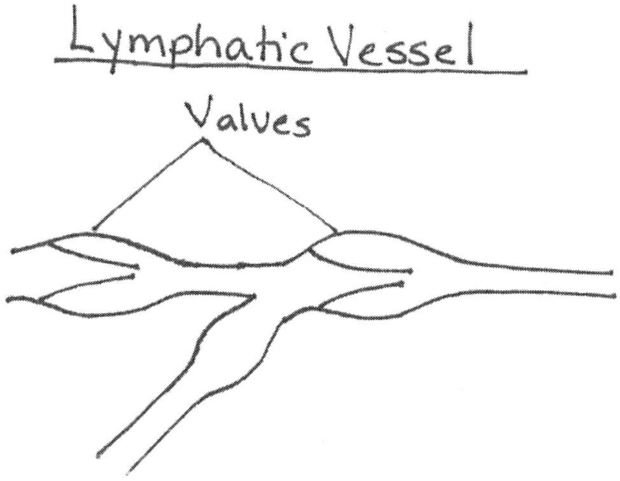

Lymphatic Vessel

Valves

There are two types of lymphatic vessels that take lymph from the lymphatic capillaries. They are the <u>superficial lymphatics</u> and <u>deep lymphatics</u>. The superficial lymphatics are found in the subcutaneous layer under the skin and in the areolar tissues of the digestive, urinary, respiratory, reproductive systems and serous membranes that line the pleural, pericardial and peritoneal cavities. Deep lymphatics are bigger and will be found near deep arteries and veins that deliver blood to the muscles and organs of the body. These guys join together to make even larger vessels called <u>lymphatic trunks</u>. The trunks empty into two collecting vessels: the <u>thoracic duct</u> and the <u>right lymphatic duct</u>. The thoracic duct grabs lymph from the area below the diaphragm and from the left side of the body above the diaphragm. The right lymphatic duct grabs lymph from the right side of the body above the diaphragm. The base of the thoracic duct is swollen and looks like a sac. It is called the <u>cisterna chyli.</u>

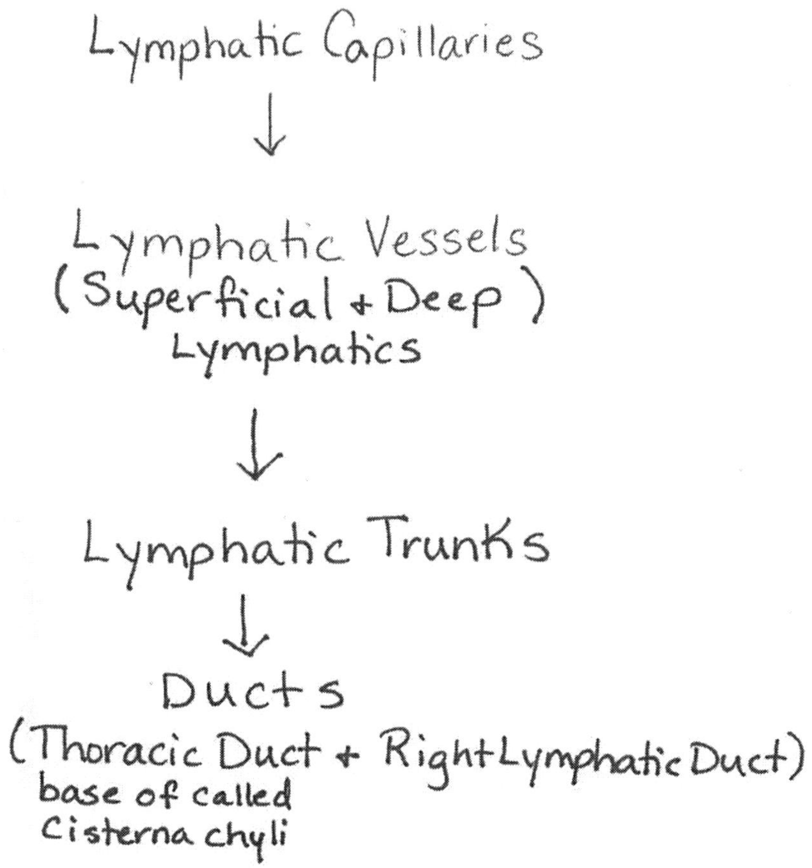

Lymphatic Capillaries

↓

Lymphatic Vessels
(Superficial + Deep)
Lymphatics

↓

Lymphatic Trunks

↓

Ducts
(Thoracic Duct + Right Lymphatic Duct)
base of called
Cisterna chyli

The cisterna chyli is located under the diaphragm (see text) and takes lymph from the lower part of the abdomen, pelvis and lower limbs. This lymph is delivered by the right and left lumbar trunks and the intestinal trunk. The thoracic duct continues upward along the left side of the vertebral column and will collect lymph near the left clavicle from the left <u>brachiomediastinal trunk, left subclavian trunk and the left jugular trunk</u> and then empties into the <u>left subclavian vein</u>. Lymph then reenters the venous circulation from the left side upper body as well as from the entire body below the diaphragm. The right lymphatic duct is formed by the union of the <u>right jugular, right subclavian and right bronchomediastinal trunks</u> near the right clavicle. This duct will empty lymph into the <u>right subclavian vein</u> delivering blood from the right side of the body above the diaphragm.

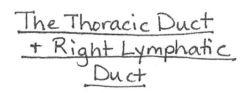

The Thoracic Duct
+ Right Lymphatic
Duct

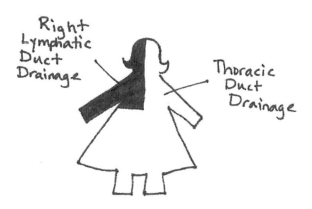

Right
Lymphatic
Duct
Drainage

Thoracic
Duct
Drainage

<u>Lymphocytes</u>

Lymphocytes can be divided into three types: 1) <u>T cells (thymus dependent)</u>, 2) <u>B cells (bone marrow derived)</u>, and 3) <u>Natural Killer (NK) cells</u>. Most lymphocytes are T cells and they can be further divided up into 4 types: <u>cytotoxic T cells, helper T cells, memory T cells, and suppressor T cells.</u>

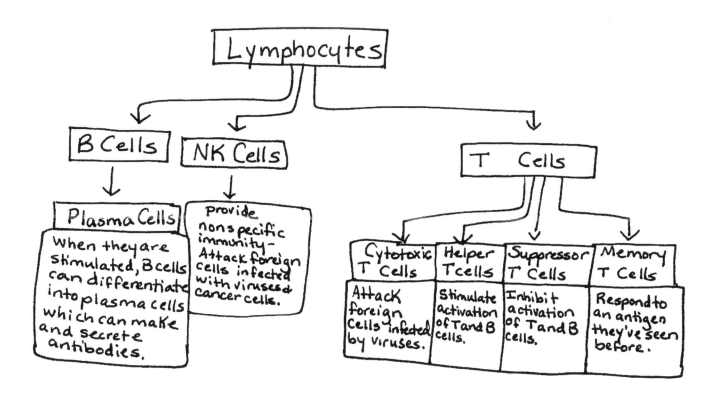

Lymphocytes

B Cells → Plasma Cells: When they are stimulated, B cells can differentiate into plasma cells which can make and secrete antibodies.

NK Cells → Provide nonspecific immunity - Attack foreign cells infected with viruses & cancer cells.

T Cells:
- Cytotoxic T Cells: Attack foreign cells infected by viruses.
- Helper T cells: Stimulate activation of T and B cells.
- Suppressor T Cells: Inhibit activation of T and B cells.
- Memory T Cells: Respond to an antigen they've seen before.

Antibodies bind to chemical targets called antigens which will start up the immune system's response. Most antigens are parts of a pathogen, the pathogen itself or a foreign substance. Antigens are usually protein but can sometimes be lipids or nucleic acids. When an antibody binds to a target antigen a chain of events will begin leading to the destruction of the target organism.

Lymphocytes move through the body. They move through tissues and will then transport themselves through the blood stream or lymphatic vessels.

Lymphocyte Production

When lymphocytes are made in the body, we call that lymphopoeisis. In lymphopoeisis we use the red bone marrow, thymus and peripheral lymphoid tissues. Red bone marrow is king of this process! Hemocytoblasts divide in the bone marrow of adults to make lymphoid stem cells that make all of the different types of lymphocytes. Two types of lymphoid stem cells are made in the red bone marrow. Some of the lymphoid stem cells stay in the red bone marrow where others migrate to the thymus. The lymphoid stem cells in the red bone marrow divide to make immature B cells and NK cells. Stromal cells in the red bone marrow are very involved in making B cells. The stromal cells have cytoplasmic extensions (kinda like tentacles) that reach out and touch or hug the developing B cells. The stromal cells make a hormone called interleukin-7 that will help encourage the differentiation of B cells. When the B cells and NK cells mature they move into the blood stream and move to peripheral tissues. The B cells move to lymph nodes, spleen or other lymphoid tissues. The NK cells or law enforcement team of the body, patrol peripheral tissues looking for abnormal cells. For the group of lymphoid stem cells that moved to the thymus, they will develop and continue to mature in seclusion. They are closed off from general circulation by the blood-thymus barrier (like blood brain barrier). The thymus makes hormones that will cause the lymphoid stem cells to divide and make the different kinds of T cells we talked about before. Once the best are selected, they re-enter the blood stream and travel to peripheral tissues.

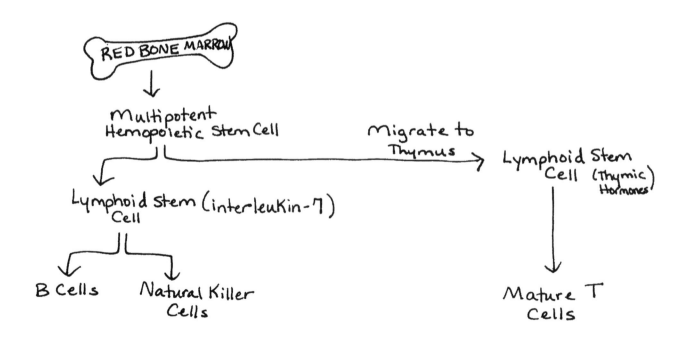

Lymphoid Organs and Tissues

Lymphoid tissues are considered connective tissues that have LOTS of lymphocytes. Along the way are lymphoid nodules which are areolar tissues that are packed to the brim with lymphocytes. A lot of times these guys are grouped together in clusters. A major example of a lymphoid nodule would be the tonsils. Inside the nodules new lymphocytes are forming.

There is a group of lymphoid tissue that protects the epithelia of the digestive, reproductive, respiratory and urinary systems. Together that group is called the mucosa-associated lymphoid tissue or MALT. (ex. Appendix)

The lymphoid organs are contained within a pouch of fibrous connective tissue to separate them from surrounding tissue. (ex. Lymph nodes, spleen and thymus) The armpits, groin and neck contain the largest amount of lymph nodes. Remember having the ones in your neck checked when you are sick? They too will protect you against infection. Lymph nodes have two types of lymphatic vessels: afferent lymphatics and efferent lymphatics. (Afferent—'A' accessing—to bring in and Efferent—'E' exiting—to take out) The afferent lymphatics bring lymph into the node from the peripheral tissues whereas the efferent brings lymph out of the node and carries it towards venous circulation. All of the lymph from the afferent lymphatics will flow through the lymph node into a subcapsular space inside the node which contains macrophages and dendritic cells which will start an immune response. Once it leaves the subcapsular space it will enter the outer cortex of the node where B cells live. It will then move through lymph sinuses in the deep cortex which is where the T cells live. The lymphocytes at this point can exit the blood stream and enter the lymph node by crossing over the wall of the blood vessel. Lymph then flows into the core (medulla) of the lymph node where more B cells and plasma cells live. The lymph then enters the efferent lymphatics. After reading through that last paragraph, doesn't a lymph node remind you of a filtration system? The lymph is cleaned before it enters the venous system. Incredibly, 99% of antigens are removed in a lymph node! The macrophages we addressed before will engulf cellular trash or pathogens. The antigens left after this process are given to lymphocytes or are bound to receptors on the surfaces of dendritic cells where they will stimulate the lymphocytes to act. This is called antigen presentation and is step one of the immune response!

The thymus is a small organ located in the mediastinum. In children it is large but after puberty it greatly decreases in size and become smaller and smaller as we age. The outer edge or cortex of the thymus contains dividing T cells which will move into the medulla once they mature. They will then leave the thymus by entering one of the blood vessels in the medulla. The lymphocytes in the cortex are surrounded by thymic epithelial cells that will monitor T cell development and function. T cells can enter or leave the bloodstream across the walls of blood vessels or through efferent lymphatics that collect lymph from the thymus.

The spleen has more lymphoid tissue than any other tissue in the body. The spleen will take abnormal blood cells and other blood parts out of the blood using phagocytosis (cellular eating). It will also start an immune response by B and T cells in response to antigen in the blood and will store iron that is recycled from blood cells. The spleen is found near the stomach and has a fibrous capsule around it as well. Inside the spleen is red pulp and white pulp. The red pulp is made of RBCs and the white pulp is made of lymphoid nodules. When blood moves through the spleen the phagocytes have an opportunity to ID and engulf damaged or infected cells in the blood. Nice filtration!

Immunity

There are two types of immunity: innate and adaptive immunity. The innate type is what you carry from your birth—you were born this way! It does not separate one threat from another. Its defense is the same no matter what is attacking your body. This type of immunity includes: physical barriers like skin, immune surveillance, phagocytic cells, interferons, inflammation, complement system and fever. The adaptive type protects you against specific threats. An adaptive defense may protect you against a particular type of pathogen but not other pathogens. These defenses develop after birth when you are accidentally or purposely exposed to an environmental hazard. B and T cells are an example of an adaptive defense. The two types of immunity work together.

Innate Defenses

The innate defenses will shield the entry or slow the spread of a microorganism. The physical barrier, such as skin, must be breached for an antigen to cause problems. Phagocytes are the cleanup crew or police in peripheral tissues. They clean up cellular trash and will respond to an invasion by a pathogen. The phagocytes include microphages and macrophages. Microphages include the neutrophils and eosinophils from the blood stream. They can leave the bloodstream and enter the peripheral tissues that may be damaged. Neutrophils are the ones that phagocytize and eosinophils will take care of the pathogens that have been coated with antibodies. Macrophages are derived from monocytes and are LARGE and very phagocytic. They can be either fixed or free meaning that fixed may stay in one place and free may migrate. Macrophages may engulf and destroy a pathogen with lysosomal enzymes, bind to or remove a pathogen from the interstitial fluid and gang up on it with other cells, or release toxic chemicals to destroy the pathogen. Free micro-and macrophages can move through a capillary wall by squeezing between the endothelial cells in the capillary. These awesome endothelial cells create markers that signal blood cells that something is wrong and then phagocytic cells migrate into the damaged tissue. Chemotaxis is when chemicals are released to attract or repel free micro-and macrophages. Also for both types of cells adhesion occurs. This is when the phagocyte attaches to the pathogen by binding to the receptors on its membrane, the cell engulfs the pathogen and then digests it. Awesome!

Macrophage

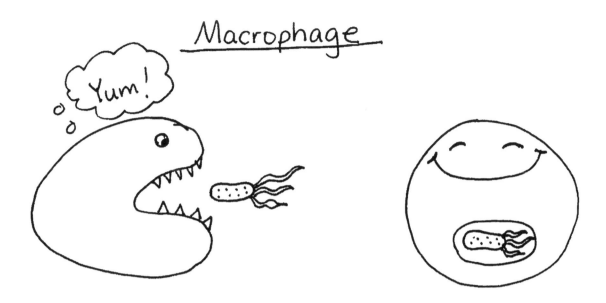

Immune Surveillance

Remember the natural killer cells or NK? They are lymphocytes that will destroy abnormal cells when they show up unannounced in the peripheral tissues. They are always watching out for these cells—that is called <u>immune surveillance</u>. When an abnormal cells arrives, it usually has foreign antigens on its surface. The NK cells will attack ANY cell with abnormal antigens (bacteria, viruses or even cancer cells). Once a NK cell is activated it will recognize the cell is not welcome and stick to the unwelcome cell. The golgi of the NK cell will then line up with the abnormal cell. The golgi then begins to spew secretory vesicles that will contain proteins called <u>perforins</u> which will be ejected by exocytosis and then will create pores in the membrane of the invader which will cause it to disintegrate.

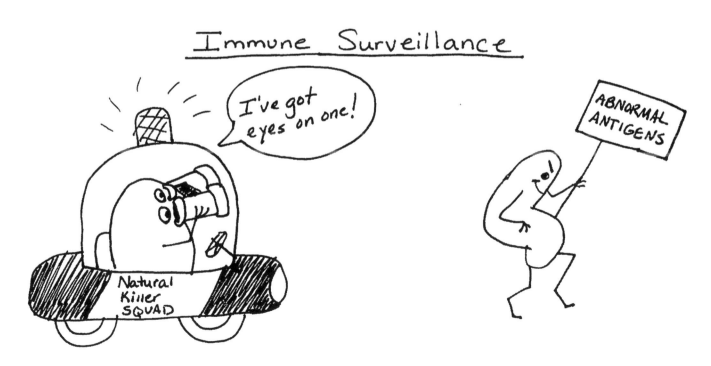

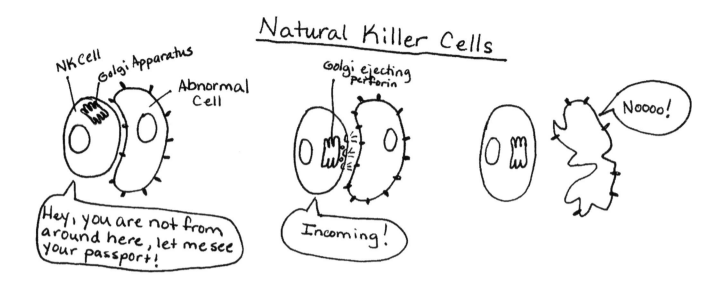

Interferons and the Complement System

Interferons or IFNs are small proteins that lymphocytes, macrophages or tissues infected with viruses release. These little guys will bind to receptors on the membranes of normal cells and using second messengers, will prompt the production of antiviral proteins in the cytoplasm of the cell. Amazingly, these proteins will mess up the process of viral replication inside the cell AND will cause the macrophages and NK cells to act. Interferon alpha, interferon beta and interferon gamma are the three types of interferon. Interferons are cytokines which act as chemical messengers that tissues release to coordinate and organize their activities. Remember paracrine communication?

In the plasma there can be found over 30 different complement or C proteins. They are all part of the complement system. These proteins will interact with each other in chain reactions. The two methods of complement activation are the classical and alternative pathway.

Inflammation and Response to Injury

Inflammation will cause the area to become red, swell, become painful and heat up. Sounds bad right? Wrong! Inflammation will cause repairs to take place and pathogens are blocked from entering the wound. It also keeps pathogens that are already in the area from spreading as easily and will send in the troops to get rid of the pathogens and start the process of regeneration.

Mast cells are largely responsible for inflammation. When an area is harmed, mast cells release histamine, heparin and prostaglandins into the interstitial fluid. Histamine will speed blood flow to the area. The increased blood flow will redden the area and make it feel warmer. Phagocyte activity increases and the raised temperature will help to denature any foreign proteins in the area. A clot will form around the damaged area to separate the area and slow down the spread of the pathogen. Complement activation through the alternative pathway will activate C3b and cause the breakdown of the bacterial cell wall. Next neutrophils move in because they are attracted in by chemotaxis. They will attack the pathogens with nitric oxide and hydrogen peroxide which they make when activated. How

Classical Pathway

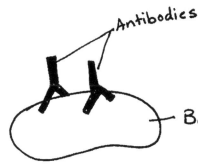

Antibodies

Bacterium

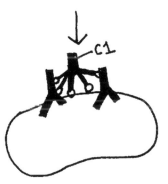

C1

- C1 is a complement protein

  C1 Attaches to
  2 antibodies

  C1 acts as enzyme, several
  reactions occur w/ other
  complement proteins.
  Inactive C3 becomes C3b
  and will attach to bacterial
  cell wall.

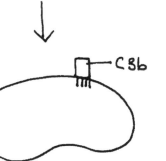

C3b

- C3b will cause: pores in
  bacterial wall + then lysis or
  attract phagocytes and make
  the bacterium easier to engulf
  OR cause mast cells to release
  histamine for inflammation
  and increase the blood flow to the
  area.

Alternative Pathway

Several complement
proteins including
Properdin interact in
the plasma in response
to bacteria and will
also result in
attachment of a
C3b protein to the
bacterial wall and
then ⌐

awesome is that? They then put out cytokines to attract other neutrophils and macrophages to the area. Fibroblasts are stimulated in by cytokines and begin forming scar tissue which will later be remodeled over time.

Fever is when your body temperature is greater than 37.2 degrees C or 99 degrees F. Your body temperature thermostat is in the hypothalamus. Proteins called <u>pyrogens</u> can reset the thermostat causing your body temperature to be raised. Pathogens or your own body cells can release these pyrogens. Fevers can be good for you within reason. The increased body temperature will slow down the spread of some bacteria and viruses and also increase the metabolic rate which will move your body's defenses much more rapidly.

<u>Adaptive Defenses</u>

The T cells and B cells are mainly in charge of adaptive defenses. These cells will respond to particular antigens. T cells will bring on <u>cell-mediated immunity</u> which will protect you against abnormal cells and pathogens and B cells will provide <u>antibody-mediated immunity</u> which will protect you against antigens and pathogens in your bodily fluids. There are different forms of immunity.

Adaptive immunity has these general properties: specificity, versatility, tolerance and memory. <u>Specificity</u> results when a specific defense is activated by a specific antigen and the response is directed at that antigen and nothing else. The shape and size of the antigen determines which lymphocyte will respond to it. Your immune system has to be ready at all times to respond to an incoming antigen. <u>Versatility</u> results because of the large diversity of lymphocytes in your body. There is a huge pool of lymphocytes with varied antigen sensitivities. This large group of lymphocytes is not enough to overcome an invasion of pathogens but when activated, a lymphocyte begins to divide making more lymphocytes with the same specificity. These cells are clones and are all sensitive to that same antigen. The immune system is not going to respond to all antigens. All cells in the body contain antigens that do not normally stimulate an immune response—the immune system exhibits <u>tolerance</u> towards those antigens. Once an immune response begins and cells have rapidly divided, two groups of cells form. One group actively attacks the pathogen, the other remains inactive unless it meets that antigen again at a later time. This group of inactive cells are called memory cells that will remember an antigen it has met before and will allow it to make a faster, stronger strike if that antigen appears again.

<u>Exploring T Cells</u>

Remember the different T cells we talked about towards the beginning of this chapter? Here's a recap: Cytotoxic T cells are in charge of cell-mediated immunity. They enter peripheral tissues and attack antigens. Memory T cells will react to antigens they have met before by making or cloning more lymphocytes to fight off the pathogen. Helper T cells stimulate the responses of both T and B cells. They have to activate the B cells to cause them to make antibodies. Suppressor T cells inhibit T and B cell activities.

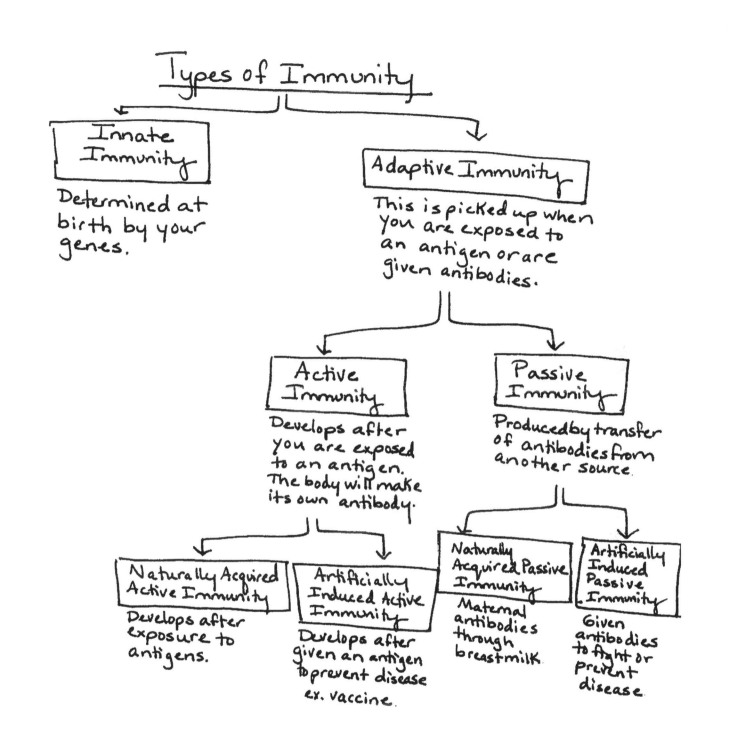

Types of Immunity

Innate Immunity
Determined at birth by your genes.

Adaptive Immunity
This is picked up when you are exposed to an antigen or are given antibodies.

Active Immunity
Develops after you are exposed to an antigen. The body will make its own antibody.

Naturally Acquired Active Immunity
Develops after exposure to antigens.

Artificially Induced Active Immunity
Develops after given an antigen to prevent disease ex. vaccine.

Passive Immunity
Produced by transfer of antibodies from another source.

Naturally Acquired Passive Immunity
Maternal antibodies through breastmilk.

Artificially Induced Passive Immunity
Given antibodies to fight or prevent disease.

For T cells to acknowledge an antigen the antigen must be bound to glycoproteins (which are part of the membrane) in the plasma membranes of another cell. When an antigen-glycoprotein combination that activates T cells appears in the plasma membrane, an antigen presentation occurs. The structure of these proteins is genetically determined. These membrane glycoproteins are called MHC (major histocompatibility complex) proteins. There are two major classes of MHC proteins—Class I and Class II. When an antigen binds to a Class I MHC protein it throws up a flag that says to the immune system, "come and destroy me!" When an antigen binds to a Class II MHC protein it says to the immune system, "I am dangerous and may hurt you—get rid of me!" Class I MHC proteins are found in the plasma membranes of all cells with nuclei. They are constantly formed and exported from the golgi. As they are forming they pick up peptides from the cytoplasm and carry them to the cell surface. If those peptides are normal the T cells ignore them but if they are abnormal or viral the T cells will become activated.

Class II MHC proteins are found in the plasma membranes of antigen-presenting cells and lymphocytes. Antigen presenting cells or APCs are cells that are in charge of activating T cell defenses against foreign cells and proteins. Phagocytic APCs engulf and then break down pathogens or foreign antigens and create fragments of the antigen which are then bound to Class II MHC proteins and put into the plasma membrane. Exposure to one of these cells can stimulate T cells.

Inactive T cells have receptors that bind Class I or Class II MHC proteins. The receptors also can bind a specific target antigen. If the protein contains any antigen other than the specific target of a particular kind of T cell, the T cell remains inactive. If the MHC protein has the antigen that the T cell is made to detect, it will bind and this is called antigen recognition—due to the fact that the T cell recognizes its target. Some T cells recognize antigens bound to Class I MHC proteins, whereas others recognize antigens bound to Class II MHC proteins. Which one a T cell responds to is dependent on the type of protein in its own membrane. These type of proteins are called CD markers. Lymphocytes and macrophages are some of the cells that have CD markers. Each of the many types of CD markers have a number. All T cells have a CD3 receptor complex in their plasma membranes—this will activate the T cell. CD8 markers are found on cytotoxic T cells and suppressor T cells –these guys respond to antigens presented by Class I MHC proteins. CD4 markers are found on helper T cells and respond to antigens presented by Class II MHC proteins.

Once a T cell has recognized an antigen it must act! It must bind to the stimulating cell at another site. This is called costimulation and confirms that the T cell should act. This is a safeguard so that the T cells don't attack normal cells. Once costimulation occurs the T cell will attack!

CD8 T Cells

There are two different types of CD8 T cells that will be activated by antigens bound to Class I MHC proteins. One will quickly make a large number of cytotoxic T cells and memory T cells and the other will slowly make a small amount of suppressor T cells. Cytotoxic T cells are the ones that will kill abnormal and infected cells. These T cells will either perforate the cell using perforin, secrete a poisonous toxin to kill it or activate genes in the infected cell's nucleus that tell the cell to die——kind of zombie-

Class I MHC Protein

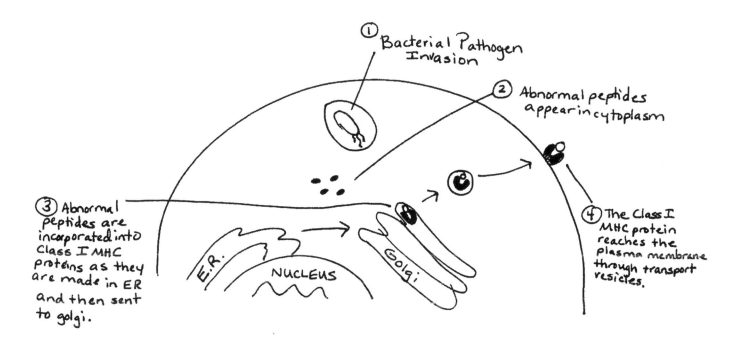

① Bacterial Pathogen Invasion

② Abnormal peptides appear in cytoplasm

③ Abnormal peptides are incorporated into Class I MHC proteins as they are made in ER and then sent to golgi.

E.R.

NUCLEUS

Golgi

④ The Class I MHC protein reaches the plasma membrane through transport vesicles.

Class II MHC Protein

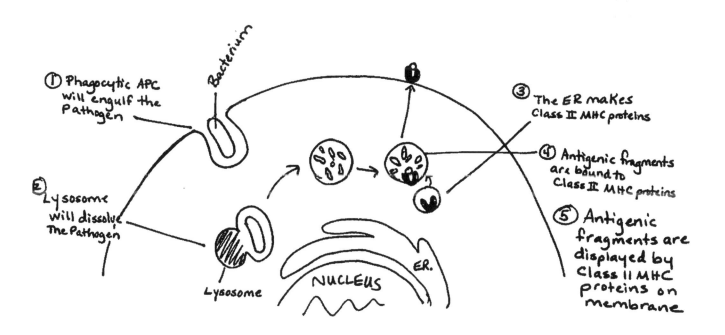

① Phagocytic APC will engulf the Pathogen

Bacterium

② Lysosome will dissolve The Pathogen

Lysosome

NUCLEUS

E.R.

③ The ER makes Class II MHC proteins

④ Antigenic fragments are bound to Class II MHC proteins

⑤ Antigenic fragments are displayed by Class II MHC proteins on membrane ish!! Memory T cells are the ones that will act when they are exposed to an antigen for the second time. They will differentiate into cytotoxic T cells. Suppressor T cells will suppress the responses of T cells and B cells by secreting inhibitory cytokines that are called suppression factors. This will help to limit the immune response from just one stimulus.

CD4 T cells

Helper T cells with CD4 markers will divide to make active helper T cells and memory helper T cells. The active helper T cells make cytokines that will push for more T cell division to make more memory helper T cells and speed up the maturation of cytotoxic T cells. The cytokines will also attract macrophages to the infected area and cause them to hang around longer and to continue active phagocytosis. They will further stimulate the activity of cytotoxic T cells and activate B cells which will lead towards the production of antibodies.

B Cells

B cells are the ones who make antibodies. B cells carry their own type of antibody in their plasma membrane. If a corresponding antigen appears in the interstitial fluid they will interact with it using these antibodies. This will activate the B cell. This is called sensitization. Remember also that B cells contain Class II MHC proteins. When sensitization happens antigens will be brought into the B cell by means of endocytosis. They will later appear on the surface of the B cells bound to Class II MHC proteins. It must receive a "go ahead" from a helper T cell (which is a safety so it doesn't overreact to an invasion). The helper T cell will bind to the B cell's MHC complex, recognize the antigen and secrete cytokines to cause the B cell to activate. The cytokines will also cause the B cell to divide and speed antibody production. When the B cell divides it will produce plasma cells and memory B cells. The plasma cells make antibodies that will have the same target as the antibodies on the surface of the parent B cell. Memory B cells remain in reserve to manage later infections that would involve the same antigens.

Antibodies

Antibodies are Y shaped molecules made of two polypeptide chains. There is one pair of heavy chains and one pair of light chains. In each chain are constant segments and variable segments. The base of the antibody molecule is made of the heavy chains. B cells make five types of constant segments. The classification scheme that identifies antibodies as IgG, IgE, IgD, IgM or IgA. How the constant segments of the heavy chain are structured determines how the antibody will be secreted and passed through the body. Some antibodies in a particular class will move in body fluids and others will bind to membranes of basophils.

The heavy chain constant segments that are bound to constant segments of the light chains, have binding sites that are covered when the antibody is first secreted. These binding sites can activate the complement system we previously talked about. When the antibody binds to an antigen, the binding sites will be uncovered. The specificity of an antibody depends on the amino acid sequence of the variable segments of the light and heavy chains. On the two variable segments there are tips called the antigen binding site. Differences in the structure of the variable segments will affect the exact shape of the antigen binding site and will make antibodies specific for different types of antigens. (See your book to view the structure of an antibody)

An antigen-antibody complex forms when an antibody binds to its corresponding antigen and is locked to it. Antibodies bind to regions on the antigen called antigenic determinant sites. The immunoglobulins or Igs are again: IgG, IgE, IgD, IgM and IgA.

IgG: the most diverse group. They help us resist bacteria, viruses and bacterial toxins. They do cross the placenta and provide passive immunity to the developing fetus.

IgE: will attach to basophils and mast cells. It causes the cell to release histamine to cause inflammation.

IgD: is also on the surface of B cells where it can bind antigens in extracellular fluid. This can help with sensitization of the B cell.

IgM: is secreted first after an antigen is met. It is responsible for the reaction in incompatible blood types and may also attack bacteria that are not affected by IgG.

IgA: found in secretions like mucous, tears and saliva. They begin attacking pathogens before they get to internal tissues.

When an antigen-antibody complex is formed, the antigen can be eliminated by a few different means. One is precipitation and agglutination. When antibodies link large numbers of antigens together, we call this an immune complex. When the antigen is a soluble molecule this process can create complexes that are too large to remain in solution—this is a precipitation. When the target antigen is on the surface of a cell or virus, the formation of these large complexes is called agglutination. Another means of elimination is neutralization. Antibodies can bind to the sites on a bacteria or virus that allow them to injure healthy cells. This would essentially keep them from attaching to the healthy cell. We can also eliminate the antigen by activation of the complement system. When an antibody binds to an antigen, parts of the antibody change shape. This will expose areas that can bind to complement proteins. This would activate the complement system. Elimination could also occur by way of opsonization. This is when antibodies and complement proteins coat the cell and make it easier for phagocytosis to occur. Antigens covered with antibodies attract eosinophils, neutrophils and macrophages for phagocytizing. Elimination could occur as well by stimulation of inflammation and also by preventing bacteria and viruses from adhering to body surfaces. This is what the dissolved antibodies in saliva, sweat and mucous do! They add an extra layer of defense.

The first immune response to an antigen is the primary response. When the antigen shows up again it will trigger a more involved and longer secondary response. This is because there is a large number of memory cells that are ready for this second arrival.

CHAPTER 22

The Respiratory System

The respiratory system is our breathing system right? Breathe in…breathe out… Yes! But it is so much more! Remember from biology how our cells must have energy to carry out all function? We make that energy using oxygen! Our circulating blood will carry oxygen from the lungs to the peripheral tissues and then the blood will transport the carbon dioxide made by the tissues back to the lungs where we can then exhale it out.

We not only use the respiratory system to move air in and out of the body, we also use it to provide a HUGE surface area to exchange the gases of carbon dioxide and oxygen. We use it to talk and also smell—the wonderful and sometimes not so wonderful olfactory sense. You can break the respiratory system down into an upper and lower portion. The <u>upper respiratory system</u> is made of the nose, nasal cavity, paranasal sinuses and the throat or pharynx. Its primary job is to filter and humidify (moisten) the air coming in. The <u>lower respiratory system</u> includes the larynx, trachea, bronchi, bronchioles and alveoli in the lungs. Its primary function is gas exchange. By the time air reaches the alveoli the air is largely filtered of particles and possible pathogens. Also, the air is humidified and ready for gas exchange.

The <u>respiratory mucosa</u> is what will line the conducting portion (entrance of nasal cavity, extending through pharynx, larynx, trachea, bronchi and larger bronchioles). The respiratory mucosa is a mucous membrane. Membranes are made of epithelial and connective tissue. Mucous membranes are made of an epithelium and layer underneath called the <u>lamina propria</u>. The lamina propria is areolar tissue and will support the epithelium of the respiratory tract. In the upper respiratory system the lamina propria contains mucous glands and in the lower respiratory system the lamina propria will contain smooth muscle.

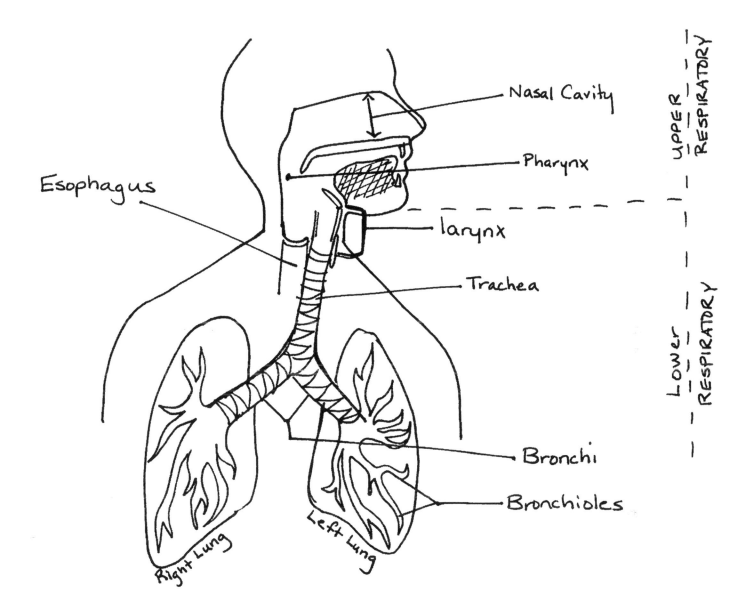

Respiratory Defense System

Our respiratory tract has a three way respiratory defense system. Ciliated epithelia line the nasal cavity and the top portion of the pharynx. It is filled with mucous cells. This mucous bathes most of the tract. The nose hairs will trap large particles. Particles that pass the nose hairs will get caught in the sticky mucous lining the pharynx, larynx, trachea and bronchi. That mucous is constantly swept by cilia towards the pharynx where it is swallowed and disposed of by stomach acid. Zap those pathogens! This is called the mucous escalator. Anything that bypasses the nose hairs and mucous escalator will meet the third line of defense, the alveolar macrophage. The alveolar macrophages patrol the alveolar surfaces and engulf foreign invaders.

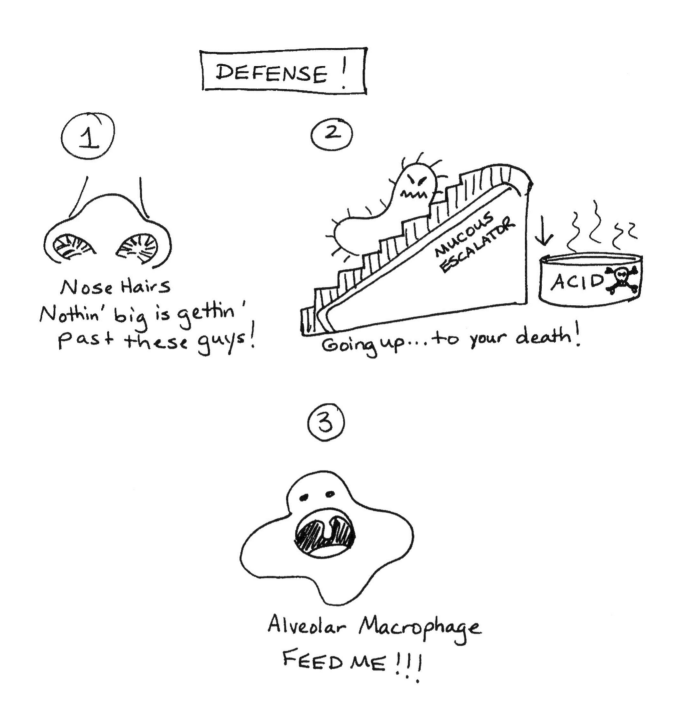

It all begins with the nose. We breathe through our nose holes/nostrils which are called the <u>external nares</u>. Here the air will first move through defense one. The nose hairs! They will trap large particles like dust and insects. Gross! The air will move into the nasal cavity which is divided into a left and right side by the <u>nasal septum</u>. This septum is made by the perpendicular plate of ethmoid and plate of vomer. Remember learning the skull? There are some bumpy things in the nasal cavity. Remember the superior, middle and inferior nasal conchae from your skull lab? They grow towards the septum from the outer walls of the nasal cavity. The air coming in will have to pass over and around and through these bumps. The passages through those bumps are called <u>superior, middle and inferior meatuses</u>. This will kick up turbulence in the air and slow it down—like speed bumps! It will help more particles be trapped in mucous and give the air extra time to be warmed and humidified. Is that awesome engineering or what? The floor of the nasal cavity is the <u>hard palate and soft palate</u>. The hard palate is made of the maxillary and palatine bone and the soft is cartilage.

The pharynx or throat is shared by the respiratory and digestive systems and can be divided into three parts: <u>nasopharynx, oropharynx and laryngopharynx</u>. The nasopharynx is connected to the nasal cavity and stops at the soft palate where the oropharynx begins. The oropharynx ends at the base of the tongue where the laryngopharynx begins. The laryngopharynx ends at the start of the larynx.

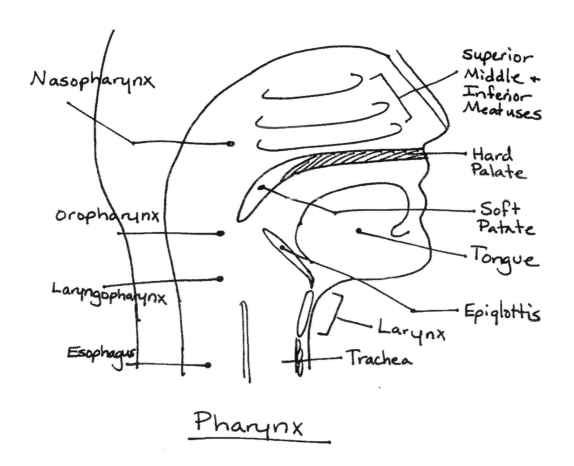

Pharynx

The air will move from the pharynx to the larynx through a little opening called the <u>glottis</u>. The glottis is our voice box! The larynx protects the glottis and is made of three large cartilages: <u>thyroid, cricoid and epiglottis</u>. The thyroid cartilage is the largest and is what you call your Adam's apple. Below it is the cricoid (reminds me of the Batman symbol). The epiglottis forms a "trash can lid" over the glottis. When you swallow saliva, food or liquids it will fold over the glottis to prevent any of those items from getting in the airway.

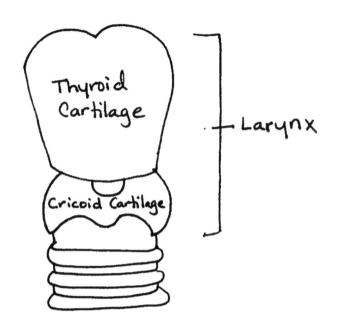

Epiglottis (Lateral/Side View)

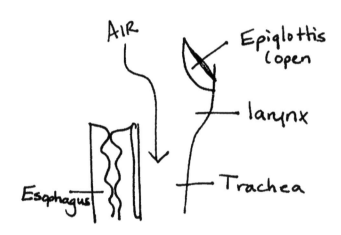

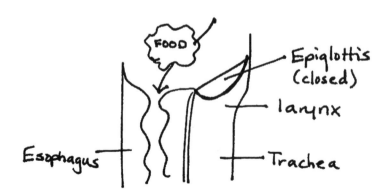

We make sounds when air passes through the glottis and vibrates the vocal folds that make it up. This produces sound waves. The pitch of the sound is determined by the width, length and tension in your vocal folds. Some of this is determined by the larynx size and some by the voluntary muscles of which you control the tension. The vocal folds of an adult male are larger than that of a female. The thicker and longer folds will produce a lower tone.

Trachea

The trachea is a tough, elastic, flexible tube that will branch to form the left and right primary bronchi. It too is coated with mucous. The trachea is held open by C-shaped tracheal cartilage rings. They are C-shaped and not closed to allow room for the esophagus to expand as food moves through.

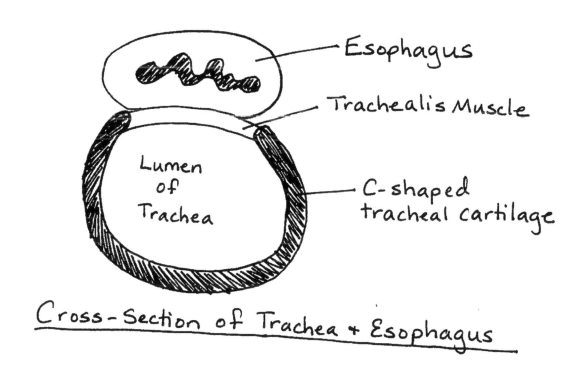

Cross-Section of Trachea + Esophagus

The mediastinum is a central tissue mass that divides the thoracic or chest cavity into a right and left pleural or lung cavity. The walls of the thoracic cavity are the ribs and the floor of it is the diaphragm. There is a serous membrane called the parietal pleura that lines the inside of the thoracic cavity. The visceral pleura covers the surfaces of the lungs. Each pleura secretes a fluid called pleural fluid. This lubricates the surfaces of the lung and thoracic cavity. It will reduce the friction between the two and prevent rubbing.

The trachea branches in the mediastinum to form the left and right primary bronchi. The bronchi enter each lung at the hilum. The hilum is a groove along the inside or medial surface of the lung where the bronchus, pulmonary (lung) vessels, lymphatics and nerves enter. The mass of items just mentioned in the previous center are enclosed within a net of dense connective tissue and is called the <u>root</u> of the lung. The lungs are made of <u>lobes</u> that are divided by deep cracks called <u>fissures</u>. The right lung is larger so it has three lobes where the left lung has two. The left lung must make room for the heart so it has a notch in it called the <u>cardiac notch</u>. The heart snuggles in here…aw!

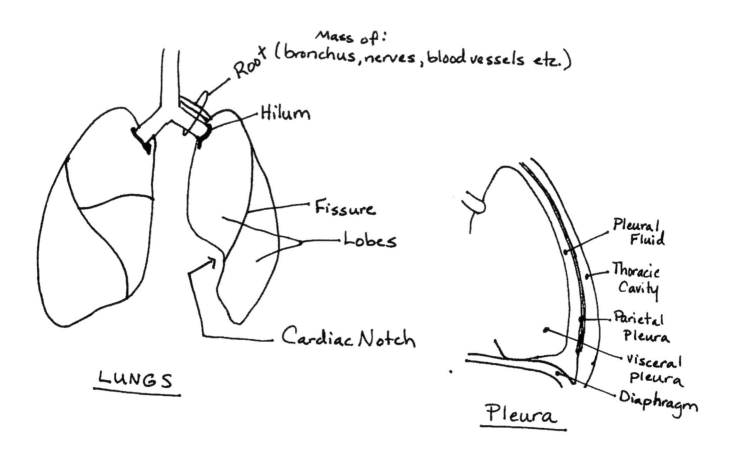

Back to the bronchi…the primary bronchi will branch into more and more fine branches—this is called the <u>bronchial tree</u>. The primary bronchi will divide to form <u>secondary bronchi</u>. One secondary bronchi goes to each lobe. The secondary bronchi divide to form <u>tertiary bronchi</u> which divide to form <u>bronchioles</u>. The bronchioles become <u>terminal bronchioles</u> and then <u>respiratory bronchioles</u>. The respiratory bronchioles are connected to individual <u>alveoli</u> and to multiple alveoli along regions called <u>alveolar ducts</u>. Alveolar ducts end at <u>alveolar sacs</u>. There are around 150 million alveoli per lung. People often picture the lungs as open hollow balloons that fill and empty with air. This couldn't be further from the truth! The 150 million alveoli give the inside of the lung a spongy appearance. It is far from hollow!

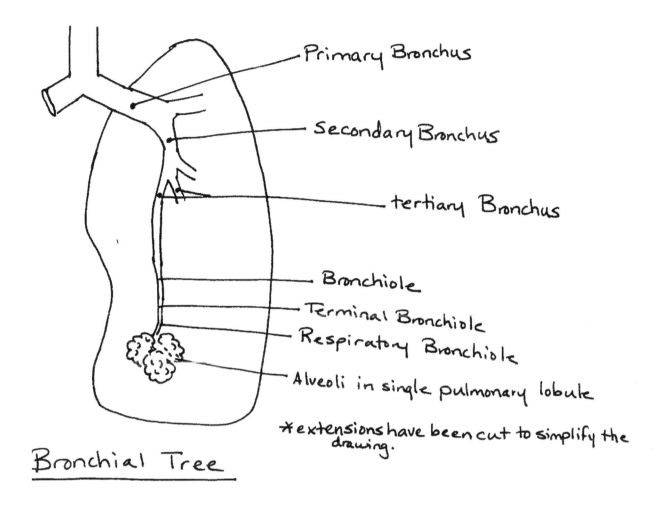

Bronchial Tree

Labels in figure:
- Primary Bronchus
- Secondary Bronchus
- tertiary Bronchus
- Bronchiole
- Terminal Bronchiole
- Respiratory Bronchiole
- Alveoli in single pulmonary lobule

✳ extensions have been cut to simplify the drawing.

Every alveolus has an amazing amount of capillaries with elastic fibers around them. These elastic fibers can recoil or squeeze during exhalation or breathing out to shrink the alveoli, pushing air out. The alveoli are mainly simple squamous epithelium. These cells are called <u>type I alveolar cells</u>. They are thin and where gas exchange happens. The alveolar macrophages we talked about earlier are patrolling these surfaces and will phagocytize any pathogens they find. <u>Type II alveolar cells or septal cells</u> are here and there throughout the squamous cells and produce <u>surfactant</u>. Surfactant is an oily secretion made of phospholipids and proteins and will coat the alveoli. It helps to keep the alveoli open by reducing surface tension. Without it the alveoli would collapse! The magic of gas exchange will happen across the <u>respiratory membrane</u> of the alveoli. The respiratory membrane is three layers: the squamous epithelial cells that line the alveolus, the endothelial cells of the capillary near the alveolus and the fused basement membranes of the alveolar and endothelial cells. In order for gas exchange to happen quickly and efficiently (who has time to wait for oxygen!?) the alveoli and capillary need to be close—I mean BEST buds. Because the alveoli and capillary are fused via their basement membranes the distance between the alveolar air and blood is only 0.5 μm. Whoa. Because of this virtually non-existent distance, the diffusion can happen almost instantaneously across the membrane.

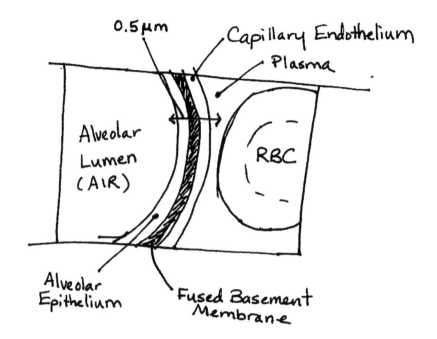

Breathing

Breathing or respiration includes <u>internal respiration and external respiration</u>. External respiration is the exchange of oxygen and carbon dioxide between the interstitial fluid and the outside of the body. Internal respiration is the absorption of oxygen and the release of carbon dioxide by those cells. We need to undergo <u>pulmonary ventilation</u>—which is fancy for breathing in and out. We need to diffuse gases across the respiratory membrane. Remember that means between the alveoli and capillaries and then between blood and the tissues of the body. Finally the transport of oxygen and carbon dioxide must occur between the alveolar capillaries and capillary beds in the body tissues.

Back to pulmonary ventilation…we want to continuously move air into and out of the alveoli. How do we move this air? The first thing we have to understand is <u>atmospheric pressure or atm</u>. Atmospheric pressure is the weight of the earth's atmosphere around us. We will move air in and out as the air pressure in the lungs moves between being below atmospheric pressure and above atmospheric pressure.

In a gas, like air, the molecules bounce around. At normal atmospheric pressure the gas molecules are farther apart and the forces acting between them are minimal. If gas is in a sealed container at atmospheric pressure the pressure exerted by the gas inside would be from gas molecules bumping into the wall of the container. More bumping equals higher pressure! If you change the volume of the container and give the gas more or less room to move around you will change the pressure.

So what the heck does all this mean?

**If volume is high, pressure is low

**If volume is low, pressure is high

When gas is in a closed container at a constant temperature, pressure (P) will be inversely proportional to volume (V). This is reciprocal. If you double the external pressure on a flexible container, its volume will drop by half. If you reduce the external pressure by half, the volume of the container will double. This relationship is called Boyle's Law.

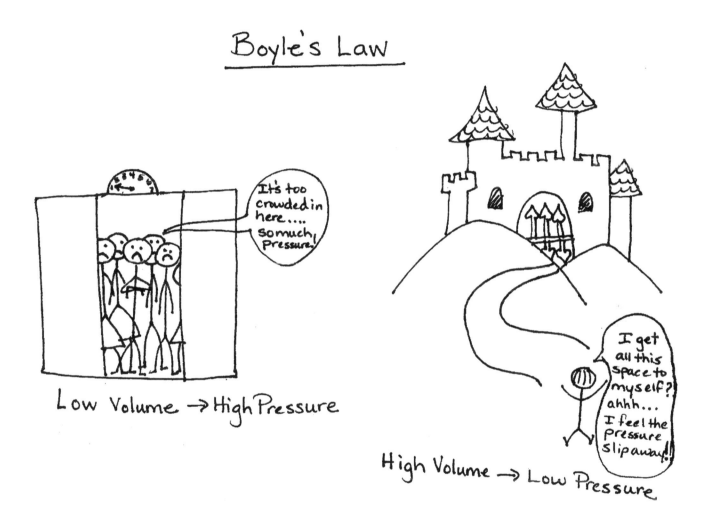

What does this have to do with breathing? Stay with me! Air will always flow from an area of higher pressure to lower pressure. One respiratory cycle will consist of an inhalation and an exhalation. The amount of air you move into or out of your lungs during a single respiratory cycle is the tidal volume. When we inhale and exhale there will be changes in the volume of the lungs which will cause differences in pressure and that will move air into or out of the respiratory system. Remember how the lungs are in a pleural cavity that is lined with a parietal pleura? Remember how the lungs are covered with a visceral pleura? Also recall that there is fluid between the parietal and visceral pleura that allow them to slide past each other?

They can slide past each other but they cannot separate under normal means because they are suctioned together. This is like:

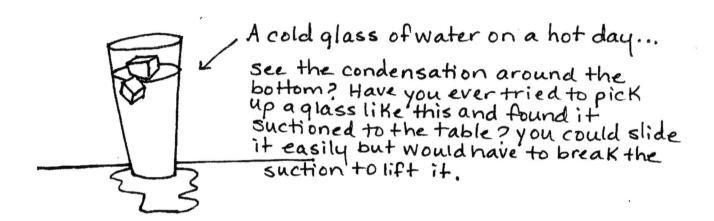

A cold glass of water on a hot day...

See the condensation around the bottom? Have you ever tried to pick up a glass like this and found it suctioned to the table? You could slide it easily but would have to break the suction to lift it.

Do you imagine that the lungs fill with air and push your chest out? Many people do but it is quite the opposite. Let's find out why...

Movements of the diaphragm or rib cage can change the volume of the thoracic cavity and will also change the volume of the lungs. The diaphragm is the floor or bottom of the thoracic cavity. It is dome-shaped. When it contracts it moves down. This will increase the volume of the thoracic cavity and decrease the pressure. (Remember if volume goes up pressure goes down) When the diaphragm relaxes, it moves up and decreases the volume of the thoracic cavity which will raise the pressure of the thoracic cavity. (If volume goes down pressure goes up) Also superior movement of the ribcage increases the depth and width of the thoracic cavity, increasing its volume. Inferior movement of the rib cage decreases the depth and width of the thoracic cavity, decreasing the volume of the thoracic cavity. When we are at rest and NOT breathing, the pressure inside and outside the thoracic cavity are equal—so no air moves in or out of the lungs. When the thoracic cavity enlarges, the lungs expand to fill that extra space. This will increase the volume and decrease the pressure inside the lungs. Air will enter because the pressure inside the lungs is lower than atmospheric pressure or pressure outside. Air will enter until the pressures inside and outside the lungs are equal. When the size of the thoracic cavity decreases, the volume of the chest cavity decreases which will raise the pressure. Air will leave the lungs because the pressure inside the lungs is greater than the pressure in the atmosphere or pressure outside.

Lung compliance is an indication of how easily they can expand. The lower the compliance the harder it is to fill the lungs—more force needed. The greater the compliance the less force needed to fill the lungs.

The direction of airflow is determined by the relationship between intrapulmonary pressure and atmospheric pressure. Intrapulmonary pressure is the pressure inside the respiratory tract at the alveoli. Intrapleural pressure is the pressure in the pleural cavity between the parietal and visceral pleurae.

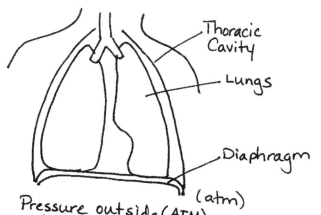

Thoracic Cavity

Lungs

Diaphragm

(atm)

Pressure outside (ATM) is equal to pressure inside thoracic cavity so no air moves.

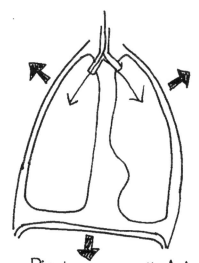

Diaphragm pulled down - increases volume of thoracic cavity. This decreases pressure inside thoracic cavity. Pressure on outside (atm) is greater than pressure inside thoracic cavity. Air moves in. Inhalation.

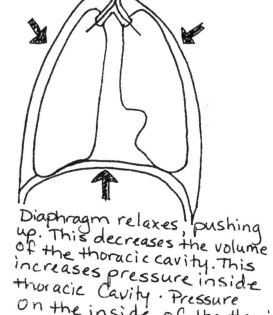

Diaphragm relaxes, pushing up. This decreases the volume of the thoracic cavity. This increases pressure inside thoracic Cavity. Pressure on the inside of the thoracic cavity is greater than outside (atm). Air moves out. Exhalation.

Types of Breathing

Eupnea or quiet breathing involves contracting the diaphragm and the external and internal intercostal muscles. Hyperpnea or forced breathing involves the diaphragm, external and internal intercostal muscles and accessory muscles.

Gas Exchange

Gases are exchanged between the alveolar air and the blood through diffusion in response to concentration gradients. The air we breathe in is a mixture of gases. The partial pressure or P of a gas is the pressure contributed by a single gas in a mixture of gases. At a given temperature, the amount of a particular gas in a solution is directly proportional to the partial pressure of that gas—this is Henry's Law. When a gas under pressure contacts a liquid, the pressure will force gas molecules into solution. The number of gas molecules rises until an equilibrium is reached. If the P of a gas increases, more gas molecules go into solution. If the P decreases, gas molecules come out of solution. Like a soda can! Soda is in a can under pressure. The gas, carbon dioxide is in solution. Once the can is open, the pressure decreases and gas begins coming out of the solution of soda. This will occur until equilibrium is reached—or your soda is flat. Gas exchange at the respiratory membrane is efficient due to the differences in partial pressure. The greater the difference in partial pressure, the faster gas will diffuse. The distance involved in gas exchange must also be short. Remember how the alveoli and capillary endothelium basement membranes were fused? We can't get closer than that! The gases must also be lipid soluble so that they can pass through the surfactant coating. We need a large surface area—which we have. There are 150 million alveoli per lung—that's a lot of surface area. Blood and airflow must also be closely coordinated.

Most of the oxygen in the blood is bound to hemoglobin or Hb on the RBCs. Hb will release the oxygen in response to changes in the partial pressure of oxygen in the plasma. If the P of oxygen is increased, Hb will bind oxygen. If the P of oxygen decreases, Hb releases oxygen. At a given P of oxygen, Hb releases more oxygen if the pH decreases. When tissues consume oxygen they generate acids that lower the pH of the interstitial fluid. When the pH decreases, the shape of the Hb molecule changes which causes the molecules to release their oxygen reserves more readily. At a given P of carbon dioxide, hemoglobin releases additional oxygen if the temperature increases. As temperature increases Hb releases more oxygen, as it decreases it holds oxygen more tightly. RBCs do not have mitochondria so they make ATP by glycolysis only. Lactic acid will be formed. Bisphosphoglycerate or BPG is also formed as a byproduct. The higher the concentration of BPG, the greater the release of oxygen by Hb molecules.

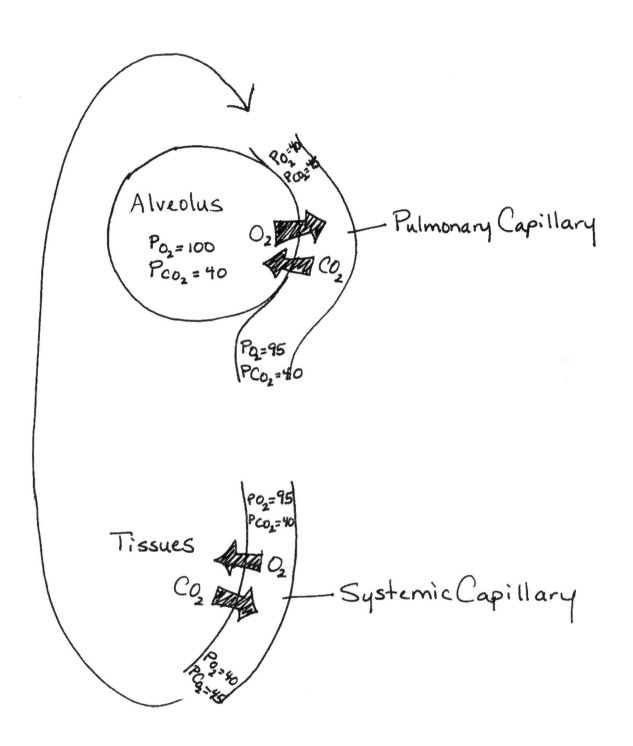

Alveolus
$P_{O_2} = 100$
$P_{CO_2} = 40$

$P_{O_2} = 40$
$P_{CO_2} = 40$

O_2

CO_2

Pulmonary Capillary

$P_{O_2} = 95$
$P_{CO_2} = 40$

$P_{O_2} = 95$
$P_{CO_2} = 40$

Tissues

O_2

CO_2

Systemic Capillary

$P_{O_2} = 40$
$P_{CO_2} = 45$

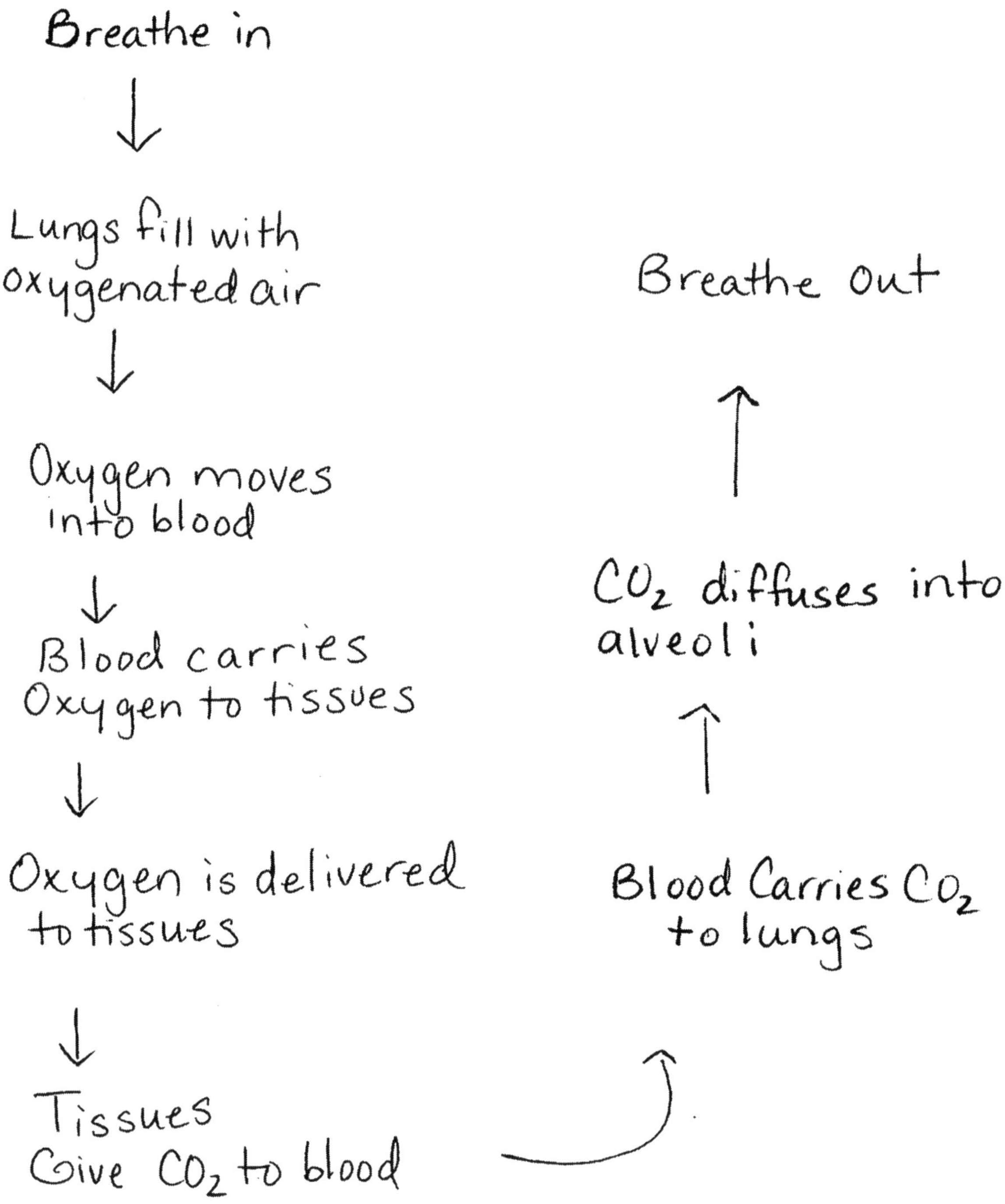

Breathe in

↓

Lungs fill with
oxygenated air

↓

Oxygen moves
into blood

↓

Blood carries
Oxygen to tissues

↓

Oxygen is delivered
to tissues

↓

Tissues
Give CO_2 to blood

Breathe Out

↑

CO_2 diffuses into
alveoli

↑

Blood Carries CO_2
to lungs

↑

Fetal Hemoglobin

Fetal Hb is different than adult Hb—it has a higher affinity for oxygen. At the same P of oxygen it binds more oxygen than does adult hemoglobin.

Carbon Dioxide Transport

Carbon dioxide is constantly generated by aerobic metabolism in the tissues. It will travel through the bloodstream in three ways.

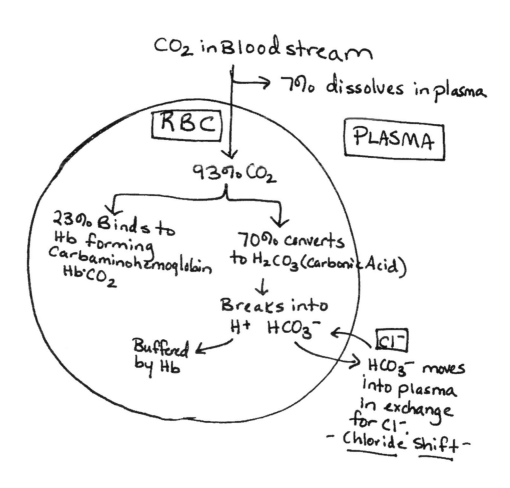

CHAPTER 23

Digestive System

We all must get nutrients from our environments so we can stay alive! Who processes and absorbs these? Why the digestive system of course! The respiratory and cardiovascular system gives us the oxygen needed for catabolism (to break things down). The digestive system works with the cardio-vascular system and lymphatic systems to give you the needed organic molecules. By using our digestive systems we are gaining the fuel that keeps our cells running and all the materials we need for cell growth and repair.

The digestive system is sometimes called the gastrointestinal or GI tract and is a long muscular tube. We begin at the oral cavity, move into the <u>pharynx, esophagus, stomach, and into the small and large intestine</u>. There are some accessory organs that help us out like the <u>teeth, tongue and glands like the gallbladder, liver, pancreas and salivary glands</u>. The food enters the GI tract and then moves along mixing with secretions and prepares for absorption into the body. Let's go through each organ step by step shall we? First we will cover the main functions of the digestive system and then we can begin to visit the parts.

<u>Ingestion</u>-In my opinion, the best part. I mean who doesn't like to eat? Especially CHOCOLATE! (I may have a problem) Sorry, anyway, ingestion is to take food into the mouth—to eat!

<u>Mechanical processing</u>—is when we crush and mash food that we just ingested—to try and make it manageable for swallowing. Imagine you could swallow an apple whole, once it made it to the stomach, it would be so difficult for the stomach to access and help to break down and harvest all of the wonderful nutrients inside. It is better, and less likely to choke you, if you break and mash the food down so that we expose more of its surface area for digestion. In this phase we use the teeth, tongue and palate. We will continue to mechanically process once we make it to the stomach and intestines.

<u>Digestion or chemical processing</u>—refers to the breakdown of food into small organic fragments that we can actually absorb across the digestive epithelium. In order to absorb these organics we must break them down into their finer components. We need to break protein down to amino acids and polysaccharides into monosaccharides for example.

<u>Secretion</u>—includes the release of water, acids, enzymes, buffers and salts by the epithelium of the GI tract and glandular organs.

<u>Absorption</u>—is where the payoff is! This is the movement of electrolytes, organic molecules, vitamins and water across the digestive epithelia and into the interstitial fluid of the GI tract.

Excretion—is the removal of wastes from the body. Wastes of the body will mix with indigestible materials and leave the body in the form of feces. The process of eliminating feces is called defecation.

Peritoneal Cavity

Inside the abdominopelvic cavity is the peritoneal cavity. The serous membrane that lines this peritoneal cavity is called the parietal peritoneum. The visceral peritoneum or serosa will cover organs that project into the peritoneal cavity. The serous membranes produce peritoneal fluid which continues to lubricate the surfaces so that the organs can slide without friction.

There are also sheets of the serous membrane that support and connect the parietal and visceral peritoneum. These are called mesenteries. They are double sheets of peritoneal membrane. In their middle they allow space for the blood vessels, nerves and lymphatics to move to and from the digestive tract. They will also help to stabilize and prevent the intestines from becoming tangled when they are squeezing and moving around during digestion. The lesser omentum is found between the stomach and the liver. I think it looks like a hammock or sling for the stomach. The falciform ligament is found between the liver and anterior abdominal wall. It helps to stabilize the position of the liver near the diaphragm and abdominal wall. There is a large pouch that originates from the stomach and hangs down in front of the intestines. This pouch is called the greater omentum and hangs like an apron. Fat can be stored in the greater omentum which can pad and protect the abdominal organs. This fat is an energy reserve, but when we store too much it gives us the apron like "beer belly." Most of the intestines are suspended by the mesentery proper. It will allow for some movement of the intestines but also stabilize them. When organs are described as retroperitoneal, this means that their bulk is behind or outside of the peritoneal cavity. The mesocolon is a type of mesentery that fuses the ascending colon, descending colon and rectum of the large intestine to the posterior body wall. These organs are retroperitoneal. The transverse mesocolon supports the transverse colon and the sigmoid mesocolon supports the sigmoid colon.

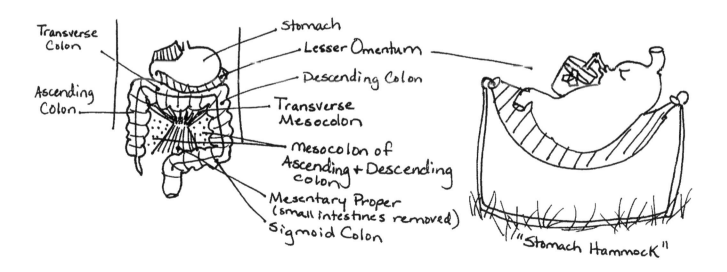

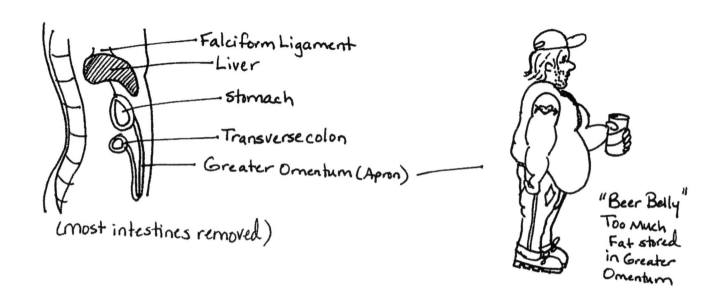

Falciform Ligament
Liver
Stomach
Transverse colon
Greater Omentum (Apron)

(Most intestines removed)

"Beer Belly"
Too Much
Fat stored
in Greater
Omentum

Histology of the Digestive Tract

If you were to take a scalpel and cut a chunk out of the wall of one of the main digestive organs you would see four main layers: <u>mucosa, submucosa, muscularis externa and serosa.</u> The details of each of these layers may differ along the tract—I'll keep you posted when that happens. Let's talk about each of those layers in more detail and then as we visit the individual organs, we will talk about their histology.

The mucosa is the innermost lining of the organ, closest to the hollow inside or lumen. It is made of epithelial tissue which is lubricated by glandular secretions. The digestive epithelium will be either simple or stratified depending on where it is. In places where abrasion is more likely, like the oral cavity, pharynx, or esophagus, stratification will be required! Have you ever accidently swallowed a chip before you finished chewing it? Ouch! In places that aren't as much in danger for mechanical damage or that are responsible for absorption like the stomach, intestines or colon, we can expect simple epithelium. These areas will also have mucous cells pumping out mucous. (To keep things nice and slippery) Scattered throughout we may also see <u>enteroendocrine cells</u> which will secrete hormones to coordinate digestion. The lamina propria is a layer of areolar tissue that contains blood vessels, nerve endings, lymphatic vessels, smooth muscle cells and lymphatic tissue. In most areas of the digestive tract, the <u>lamina propria</u> contains a sheet of smooth muscle and elastic fibers called the <u>muscularis mucosae</u>. These smooth muscle cells are layered in two concentric layers. The inner layer circles the lumen (circular muscle) and the outer layer has muscle cells arranged parallel to the long axis of the digestive tract (longitudinal layer). Contractions in these layers will move the epithelial folds. This movement will become important later!

The submucosa is made of dense irregular connective tissue and is found below the mucosa. It binds the mucosa to the muscularis externa. The submucosa is very vascular—lots of blood vessels—and also lymphatic vessels. In some areas of the digestive or GI tract, the submucosa has exocrine glands that will secrete buffers and enzymes into the lumen of the digestive tract. It also contains a network of nerve fibers and neurons called the submucosal plexus. These sensory neurons, sympathetic and parasympathetic connections, will control the mucosa and submucosa. Parasympathetic or "rest and digest" will increase muscle activity in the GI tract, whereas sympathetic stimulation will decrease muscle activity in the GI tract.

The muscularis externa is dominated by smooth muscle cells. These cells are also layered in an inner circular layer and outer longitudinal layer. When these guys activate and squeeze, this will help with mechanical processing and moving things along the tract.

The serosa is a serous membrane that covers the muscularis externa in most digestive organs of the tract. In the oral cavity, pharynx, esophagus and rectum a dense network of collagen called the adventitia attaches the digestive tract to a nearby structure.

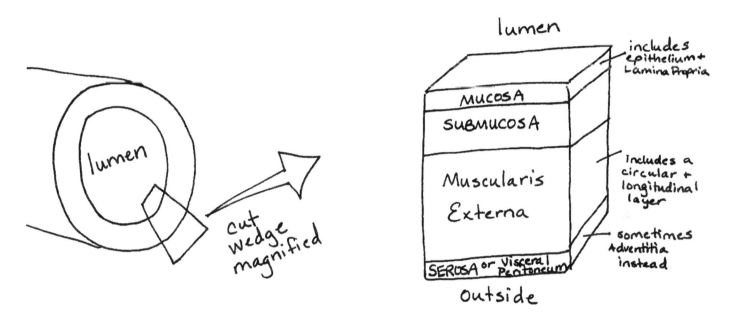

Types of Digestive Movement and Control

The smooth muscle along the digestive tract has pacesetter cells that will keep a rhythmic cycle of activity in the muscle. These cells will allow for spontaneous depolarization which will start a wave through the entire layer of muscle. These pacesetter cells are located in the muscularis mucosae and muscularis externa. They are responsible for peristalsis and segmentation. The muscularis externa will move materials from one part of the digestive tract to another by contractions called peristalsis. Peristalsis motions are wave-like. These wave like motions will move a bolus (small oval mass of digestive contents) along the length of the GI tract. Peristalsis motions are much like when you squeeze toothpaste out of a tube. Your hand is like the muscle forcing the toothpaste or bolus out of the tube or digestive tract. Segmentation is more of a churning or chopping motion. During segmentation we are mixing the contents with intestinal secretions. We are not really moving the digested contents, we are trying to further mechanically break and mix them up.

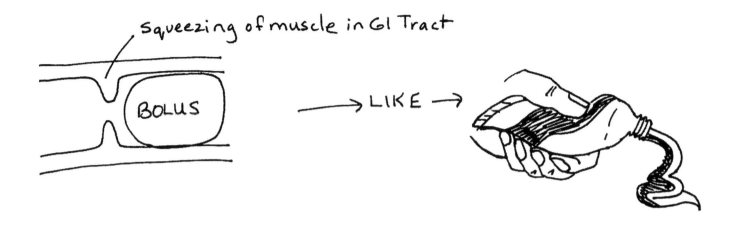

Squeezing of muscle in GI Tract

BOLUS → LIKE →

Regulation of the digestive functions begin first at the <u>local level</u>. Changes in pH, volume or the chemical composition of the tract's contents can have a direct effect on digestive activity in that part of the GI tract. Stretching of the walls of the intestines or stomach can stimulate contraction in smooth muscle or the release of chemicals that aid in digestion. <u>Neural mechanisms</u> are next. They control digestive tract movement. Sensory receptors in the walls of the GI tract can trigger peristalsis that is limited to a small area. These reflexes control localized activities that will involve only short segments of the GI tract. <u>Hormonal Mechanisms</u> can enhance or inhibit the sensitivity of smooth muscle to neural commands. These hormones will be mentioned as we move along the section of the tract.

<u>The Oral Cavity</u>

It all begins at the oral cavity, also known as the <u>buccal cavity</u>. Again, this is the BEST part of digestion in my view! This is where we analyze the food… Is it hot? Cold? Salty? Sour? Sweet? Is it chocolate—then I love it! We mechanically process the food using the teeth, tongue and palate. In other words we smash it up to make it manageable for swallowing. We lubricate it with mucous and saliva and we begin the breakdown of carbohydrates and lipids. The oral cavity is lined with mucosa that is stratified. The hard and soft palates are the roof of the oral cavity and the tongue makes up the floor of the oral cavity. The tongue pushes the food around and compresses it into a bolus. It also has the lovely sense of taste AND it releases an enzyme called <u>lingual lipase</u>. Lingual lipase will start the digestion of lipids. The tongue has two groups of skeletal muscles: the <u>intrinsic and extrinsic</u>. The intrinsic muscles will change the shape of the tongue, like when you talk. The extrinsic muscles will perform all main movements of the tongue. The salivary glands will secrete saliva into the oral cavity. There are 3 pairs of salivary glands. The <u>parotid glands</u> are in front of the ears and produce a saliva that contains large amounts of <u>salivary amylase</u> which breaks down starches (complex carbohydrates). The sublingual glands are under the tongue and produce a mucous secretion that will behave as a buffer and a lubricant. The <u>submandibular glands</u> are under the jaw or mandible and make a mixture of buffers, glycoproteins called <u>mucins</u> and salivary amylase. Saliva is mostly water but also contains electrolytes like Na^+, buffers, glycoproteins, antibodies and enzymes. The glycoproteins called mucins are what give saliva its lubricating abilities. Saliva helps to keep your mouth clean and to keep your mouth at a pH of around 7.0.

The teeth are also super critical to the process of mechanical processing. The tongue will help to push food into the occlusal or opposing surfaces of the teeth. Chewing or mastication will occur. The bulk of each tooth is made of a dense mineral substance called dentin. The tooth has blood vessels and nerves in it and sits in a socket called the alveolus. The periodontal ligament holds it into the socket. The crown is the exposed surface of the tooth and is covered with enamel. Enamel is SUPER hard and resists decay. There are four main types of teeth: incisors, cuspids or canines, bicuspids or premolars and molars. Incisors are blade-shaped teeth and are great for clipping or cutting and have a single root. Cuspids or canines are cone-shaped and are better for tearing and have a single root. Bicuspids or premolars have flattened crowns with high ridges. They are good at crushing and grinding and typically have one or two roots. Molars are larger with flattened crowns and they excel at crushing and grinding and typically have two to three roots. You have two sets of teeth in life: deciduous teeth or the temporary teeth of primary dentition and the secondary dentition or permanent teeth. The deciduous teeth or primary dentition are what we often call baby teeth. Most children have 20. The secondary dentition or permanent teeth of adults are numbered at 32.

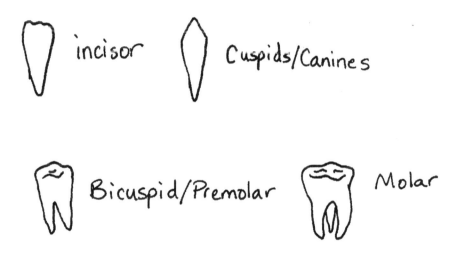

The Pharynx

The pharynx, also known as the throat, will allow for the passage of food, liquids and air. Remember that there is a naso-, oro- and laryngo-pharynx? The pharynx is mostly lined with stratified squamous epithelia. We will also find mucous glands and some lymphatic tissue in the tonsils. The pharynx has some muscles that will help us with the process of swallowing or deglutition. The pharyngeal constrictor muscles push the bolus toward the esophagus. The palatopharyngeus and stylopharyngeus muscles elevate the larynx and the palatal muscles elevate the soft palate and nearby parts of the pharyngeal wall. These muscles team up with the muscles of the oral cavity and esophagus to start swallowing which will push the bolus into the esophagus, through it, and finally towards the stomach.

The Esophagus

The esophagus is a hollow muscular tube that will bring solid food and liquids to the stomach. It passes through an opening in the diaphragm called the esophageal hiatus.

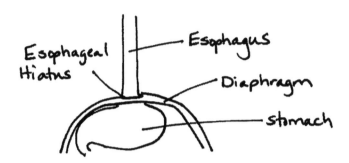

The histology of the esophagus contains mucosa, submucosa, muscularis externa and adventitia. The mucosa is made of stratified squamous epithelia and is packed into large folds that will allow for expansion of the esophagus when a bolus passes through. The muscularis mucosae is made of an irregular layer of smooth muscle. The submucosa has esophageal glands that make mucous to help lubricate it so that the bolus can move smoothly through. The muscularis externa is made of the inner circular and outer longitudinal layers. There is also skeletal muscle throughout. This is so that swallowing can be under conscious control. You can decide if you want to drink or swallow food right? Yep! Skeletal muscle is voluntary! You do swallow when you aren't thinking about it too right? Yep again! Smooth muscle is involuntary. There is no serosa but an adventitia instead.

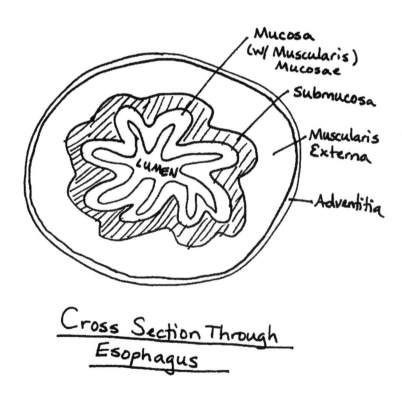

Cross Section Through Esophagus

Swallowing or deglutition is initiated under our conscious control but proceeds involuntarily once it begins. The swallowing reflex begins when receptors on the palatal arches and uvula (that little punching bag thing in your throat) are stimulated by the bolus. This information is passed to the swallowing center of the medulla oblongata. This will trigger the pharyngeal musculature. The bolus will be pushed into the esophagus. Your breathing will stop. We can divide this into three phases: buccal, pharyngeal and esophageal.

In the buccal phase we will compress the bolus against the hard palate and then force the bolus towards the oropharynx. The soft palate will elevate and seal off the nasopharynx. In the pharyngeal phase the bolus moves through the oropharynx and the larynx elevates. When the larynx elevates the epiglottis will close over the glottis. In the esophageal phase the pharyngeal muscles force the bolus through the entrance to the esophagus. Once it enters the esophagus it will be pushed toward the stomach via peristalsis. When the bolus reaches the lower esophageal sphincter, it will open and allow the bolus to enter the stomach.

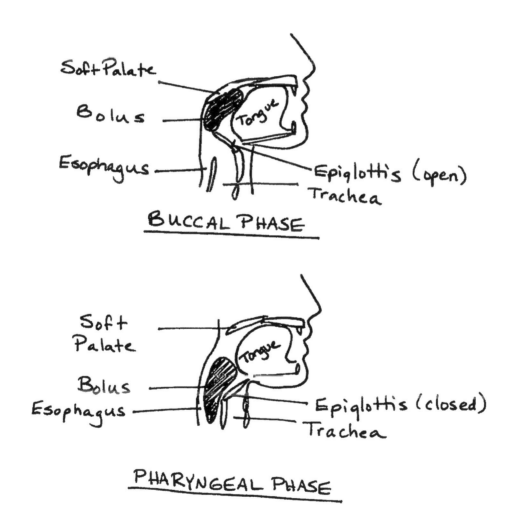

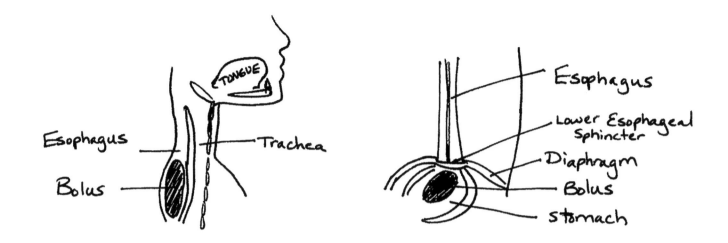

ESOPHAGEAL PHASE

The Stomach

The stomach will store undigested food, help to mechanically process the food, chemically break down the food using acids and enzymes and it will produce intrinsic factor. Intrinsic factor is a glycoprotein your body needs to absorb vitamin B_{12} in the small intestine. Once the bolus enters the stomach it combines with mucous, acids and enzyme to form an acidic mixture called chyme. The stomach is muscular and J-shaped. At its end there is a pyloric sphincter that will allow it to empty into the duodenum. The stomach's volume expands and shrinks as it fills and empties. The stomach has extra tissue for expansion called rugae. These wrinkles of extra tissue are found lining the stomach wall.

The histology of the stomach contains a mucosa, submucosa, muscularis externa and serosa. The mucosa is made of simple columnar epithelia that produces mucous that covers the lining of the stomach. This mucous will protect the stomach from its own acid and enzymes. There are shallow pits in the mucosa called gastric pits. At the base of the pit are mucous cells. In some parts of the stomach a single gastric pit communicates with several gastric glands which dip deep down into the lamina propria. Gastric glands have two types of secretory cells: parietal and chief cells. Together they secrete gastric juice. Parietal cells secrete intrinsic factor and hydrochloric acid or HCl. This HCl will keep the stomach contents at a pH of 1.5-2.0. This acidity will kill most microorganisms that are ingested with food. It will also help to break-down or denature proteins, break down plant cell walls, meat and finally activate pepsin. Pepsin is an enzyme that helps to digest protein. Chief cells secrete pepsinogen which is inactive and will convert to pepsin when exposed to acid. Glands in the pylorus, called pyloric glands, produce a mucous secretion. There are also cells called enteroendocrine cells. One of the hormones they produce is gastrin which is produced by the G cells. Gastrin will stimulate secretion of the parietal and chief cells and cause contractions of the stomach wall to mix things up. There are also D cells that make somatostatin, a hormone that inhibits the release of gastrin.

Histology of The Stomach

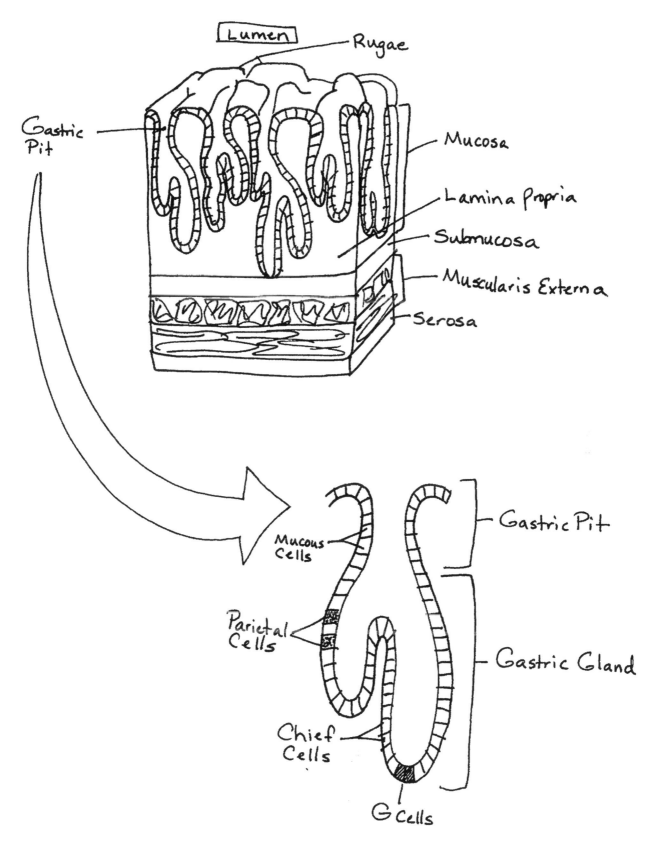

Lumen

Rugae

Gastric Pit

Mucosa

Lamina Propria

Submucosa

Muscularis Externa

Serosa

Mucous Cells

Gastric Pit

Parietal Cells

Gastric Gland

Chief Cells

G Cells

The production of acids and enzymes by the stomach can be controlled by the CNS, the nerves in the digestive tract or by hormones of the digestive tract. Here are the three overlapping phases:

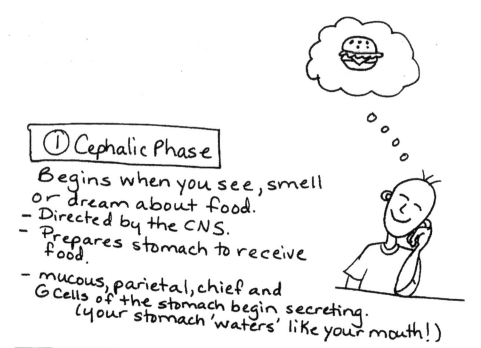

① Cephalic Phase

Begins when you see, smell or dream about food.
- Directed by the CNS.
- Prepares stomach to receive food.
- mucous, parietal, chief and G cells of the stomach begin secreting. (your stomach 'waters' like your mouth!)

② Gastric Phase

Begins when food arrives in stomach.
- Stretching of the stomach, increase in pH + the entry of undigested materials (like proteins) will initiate this phase.

   3 mechanisms occur!

- **Local Response** – stretching of stomach wall causes release of histamine which stimulates parietals cells and causes them to release acid.
- **Neural Response** – stretch and chemical receptors activate secretory cells and makes powerful mixing waves in stomach wall.
- **Hormonal Response** - neural stimulation and presence of peptides and amino acids in chyme cause release of gastrin, which causes parietal and chief cells to secrete. this reduces pH + stimulates gastric motility.

③ Intestinal Phase

Begins when chyme enters small intestine.
- Once chyme leaves stomach and enters duodenum this triggers receptors that will trigger a reflex that stops gastrin production and contractions.

The stomach will allow preliminary digestion of protein by pepsin. There is virtually no absorption of nutrients here due to the blanket of mucous and also digestion is not finished!

Small Intestine

This is where chemical digestion will be completed and we can absorb 90 percent of nutrients! Finally! The small intestine has three regions: duodenum, jejunum and ileum. The duodenum is only about 25 cm long and is sometimes called the mixing bowl of the small intestine because secretions of the liver, gall bladder and pancreas mix with the chyme here. The jejunum is about 2.5 meters long and is where the bulk of chemical digestion and nutrient absorption happen. The ileum is the last segment of the small intestine and is the longest at 3.5 meters long. The ileum empties into the large intestine at the ileocecal valve.

The histology of the small intestine also includes mucosa, submucosa, muscularis externa and serosa. The mucosa has folds in it that are permanent called plicae. These are part of what greatly increases the surface area of the small intestine for absorption. The plicae are also covered with fingerlike projections called villi which are further covered by microvilli! Without the plica, villi and microvilli the small intestine would only have area of 3300 cm² to absorb across. WITH the plicae, villi and microvilli we have 2 million cm² of area to absorb across.

The lamina propria has a large network of capillaries that come out of a larger network in the submucosa. These capillaries carry freshly absorbed nutrients to the hepatic portal circulation for delivery to the liver. The liver will adjust the nutrient concentration of the blood before it reaches the general circulation. Each villus also has a lymphatic capillary called a lacteal. Lacteals will transport materials that are not able to enter the blood capillaries. Fatty acids are packaged into protein-lipid combos that are too large to move into the bloodstream. These guys are called chylomicrons. They will eventually reach the venous circulation. The epithelia lining the small intestine is simple columnar. Between the simple columnar cells are mucous cells that eject mucins onto the intestinal surfaces. There are also intestinal glands that extend deep into the lamina propria. One of the most important enzymes formed and pushed into the lumen are called brush border enzymes. These are proteins on the surface of microvilli that break down materials that come in contact with the microvilli and then absorb the broken down products. Intestinal glands also contain enteroendocrine cells that release the hormones gastrin, secretin and cholecystokinin. Glands in the duodenum called duodenal glands are responsible for creating excess mucous to protect the duodenum from acids normal for the stomach. They also secrete a hormone called urogastrone that is responsible for inhibiting gastric acid production and will stimulate division of stem cells in the epithelia of the digestive tract. In the ileum we will find Peyer's patches which are lymphoid nodules that protect the small intestine from bacteria that are normal for the large intestine.

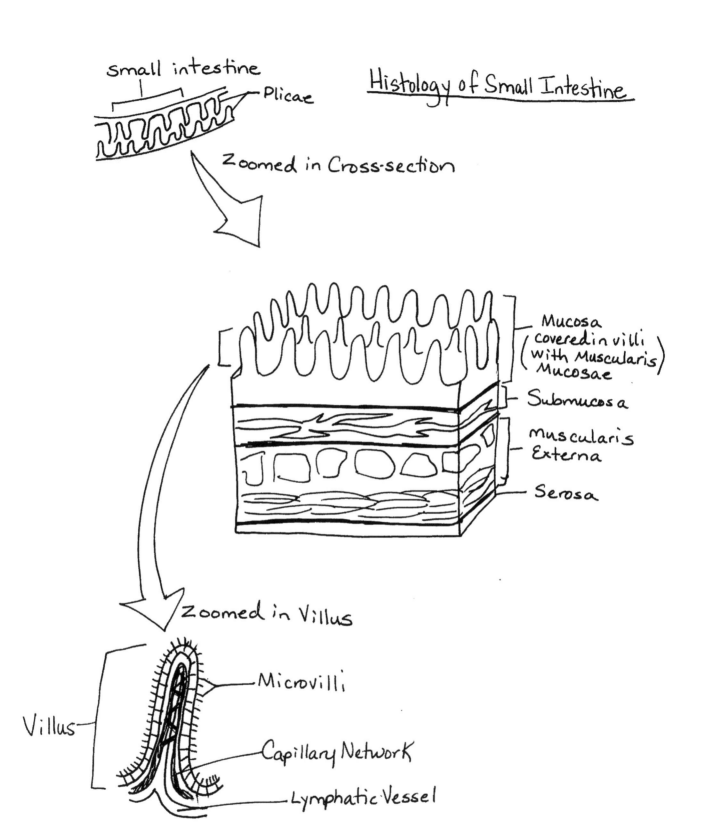

small intestine

Plicae

Histology of Small Intestine

Zoomed in Cross-section

Mucosa
(covered in villi
with Muscularis)
Mucosae

Submucosa

Muscularis
Externa

Serosa

Zoomed in Villus

Microvilli

Capillary Network

Lymphatic Vessel

Villus

After chyme has arrived in the duodenum, weak peristalsis moves it slowly towards the jejunum.

The Pancreas

The pancreas is below the stomach and very close to the duodenum. It is mostly exocrine and makes digestive enzymes and buffers. These secretions are delivered to the duodenum by the pancreatic duct. The common bile duct also delivers secretions here. The pancreas secretes pancreatic juice, which is an alkaline mixture of digestive enzymes, water and ions, into the small intestine. This is going to break things down to the level that we can absorb them. Cholecystokinin will stimulate the production and secretion of pancreatic enzymes. The first pancreatic enzyme is a carbohydrase—an enzyme that breaks down certain starches or carbohydrates. The next pancreatic enzyme is lipase that will breakdown certain lipids. Another pancreatic enzyme is nuclease which will break down RNA or DNA. Finally there are the proteolytic enzymes that will break apart certain proteins.

The Liver

It is the hub of metabolic regulation in the body. It is large, firm and reddish brown. The liver is wrapped in a tough fibrous capsule and is made of liver cells called hepatocytes. The hepatocytes adjust circulating levels of nutrients through selective absorption and secretion. The liver is divided into 100,000 lobules by connective tissue. The hepatocytes in a lobule form a series of plates arranged much like a wagon wheel. As blood flows through the liver, hepatocytes absorb solutes from the plasma and secrete materials like plasma proteins. The liver secretes bile into a network of narrow channels called bile canaliculi which will connect to bile ductules and then to the bile ducts. The right and left hepatic ducts collect bile from all the bile ducts of the liver lobes and then combine to form the common hepatic duct. The bile in the common hepatic duct flows into the common bile duct and the cystic duct which empties into the gall bladder.

The liver is involved in regulating circulating blood. All blood that leaves the absorptive area of the digestive tract enters the liver. The liver is part of your metabolic regulation. Liver cells extract nutrients or toxins from the blood before it reaches general circulation. It will remove and store excess nutrients. The liver stabilizes blood glucose. If blood glucose is low, hepatocytes will break down stored glycogen in the liver and release glucose into the blood. The liver can also make glucose from other carbohydrates. The liver also regulates levels of triglycerides, fatty acids and cholesterol. The liver removes excess amino acids from the bloodstream, helps with waste product removal, vitamin storage, mineral storage, and drug inactivation.

The liver assists in hematological regulation. As blood passes through it, cells in it will engulf old or damaged red blood cells, pathogens and cellular debris, removing them from the bloodstream. The liver cells make and release most of the plasma proteins like albumin. It will also remove circulating hormones like epinephrine, insulin and steroid hormones. It removes antibodies and breaks them down, releasing amino acids for recycling. It will remove toxins in the diet and make bile which will help us to digest lipids.

Most lipids we ingest are not water soluble. When they mix in the stomach large drops are created that contain a variety of lipids. Bile salts break down these large drops in a process called <u>emulsification</u>. Emulsification will allow an increased surface area for enzymes to act on these lipids. After lipid digestion has been completed, bile salts will promote the absorption of lipids with the intestinal epithelium. The majority of bile salts themselves will also be absorbed. The reabsorbed bile salts enter the hepatic portal circulation and then they are recycled.

<u>Gallbladder</u>

The gallbladder is a hollow pear-shaped organ that stores and concentrates bile. The major function of the gallbladder is bile storage, but it is released into the duodenum only under the stimulation of the intestinal hormone cholecystokinin or CCK. When CCK is released, this will cause contractions of the gallbladder that will push bile into the small intestine—especially when there are large amounts of lipids.

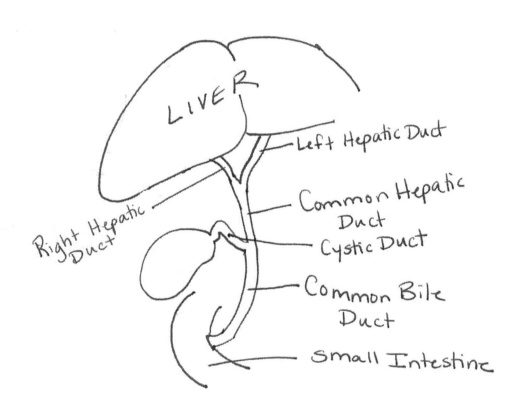

On average it takes about five hours for materials to pass from the duodenum to the ileum.

Large Intestine

The large intestine begins at the ileum and ends at the anus. It frames the small intestine like a picture frame. The main function is to store digestive wastes and reabsorb water. Bacteria that live in the large intestine are a great source of vitamins like vitamin K, biotin and vitamin B_5. The large intestine can be divided into three parts, the cecum, the colon and the rectum.

The cecum begins after the ileocecal valve. It begins the process of compaction. The appendix is attached to the cecum. The colon has pouches called haustra which allow the colon extra expansion. The colon includes the ascending, transverse, descending and sigmoid. The rectum temporarily stores feces. The movement of fecal material into the rectum triggers the defecation reflex.

Histology and Function of the Large Intestine

The colon does not have villi. There are lots of mucous cells and intestinal glands. The mucous provides lubrication as the fecal material becomes drier and more compact. The reabsorption of water is huge in the large intestine. The bacteria that live in the large intestine will generate three vitamins that are critical for our diets. Vitamin K is a vitamin the liver needs to make four clotting factors for blood clotting. Biotin is important in the aid of glucose metabolism. Vitamin B_5 is needed to make steroid hormones and some neurotransmitters. Organic wastes are important to get rid of. In the large intestine, bacteria convert bilirubin to urobilinogen and stercobilinogen. Some urobilinogens are absorbed into the bloodstream and then excreted in urine. The urobilinogen and stercobilinogens remaining in the colon are converted to urobilins and stercobilins by being exposed to oxygen. These are what give feces a yellow-brown color. Bacteria also break down peptides that are in the feces which creates ammonia, nitrogen containing compounds that contribute to the odor of feces and hydrogen sulfide (a gas with a rotten egg odor). Powerful peristaltic contractions or mass movements in the colon happen a few times a day. Distention of the rectal walls will trigger the defecation reflex. Both the internal and external anal sphincters must relax for feces to be eliminated.

A healthy diet contains everything you need to maintain homeostasis. These main ingredients of health are: carbohydrates, lipids, proteins, vitamins, minerals and water.

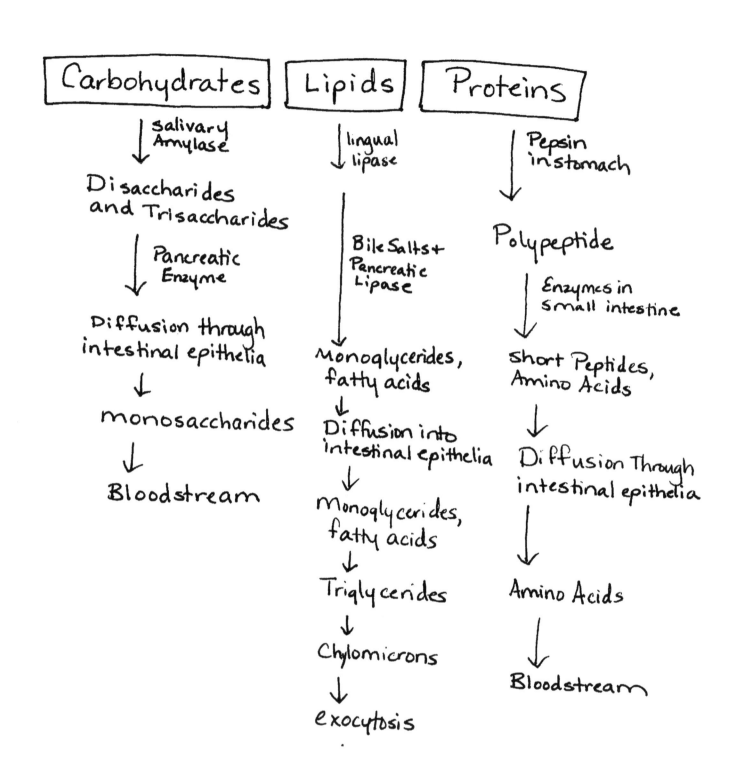

CHAPTER 24

The Urinary System

The urinary system has three major functions: excretion of organic waste products from the body fluids, elimination of this waste into the outside world and regulation of the homeostasis of the volume and solute concentration of the blood. The organs involved in this are the kidneys, ureters, bladder and urethra. The kidneys produce urine which is carried to the bladder for storage by the ureters. The urethra will carry the urine to the outside of the body. The urinary system removes wastes made by the cells in the body but also has some other important functions. These include regulation of blood volume and pressure, regulation of plasma concentrations of sodium, potassium, chloride and other ions, stabilizing blood pH, conserving nutrients and assisting the liver in the detoxification process. You can kinda look at the kidneys as a blood filtration system!

The kidneys are often a lot higher in the body than people think. They are partially enclosed in the ribcage. On top of the kidneys lie the adrenal glands. The kidneys are retroperitoneal which means they lie behind or outside of the peritoneal cavity. The fibrous capsule covers the kidney, which is surrounded by a layer of fat called the perinephric fat, and then coated by renal fascia. The renal fascia is a fibrous outer layer that anchors the kidney to surrounding structures. The hilum is an indentation in the kidney where the renal artery, renal vein and the ureter enter the kidney.

The kidney has an outer cortex and an inner medulla. The cortex is the outer portion of the kidney. The renal medulla is made of 6-18 renal pyramids. The wide part of the pyramid touches the cortex. The pointy part of the pyramid is called the renal papilla. Bands of tissue from the cortex separate the pyramids and are called the renal columns. A kidney lobe is made of a renal pyramid, the renal cortex on top of it and the adjacent renal columns. Urine is made in these lobes. Ducts within each renal papilla will drain urine into a cup shaped drain called a minor calyx. Four or five minor calyces join to form a major calyx and two or three major calyces join to form the renal pelvis. The renal pelvis joins to the ureter where urine is drained down to the urinary bladder.

The kidneys are very vascular. The renal artery delivers blood to the kidney and branches into finer and finer vessels where the blood is filtered. The renal vein takes blood out of the kidney.

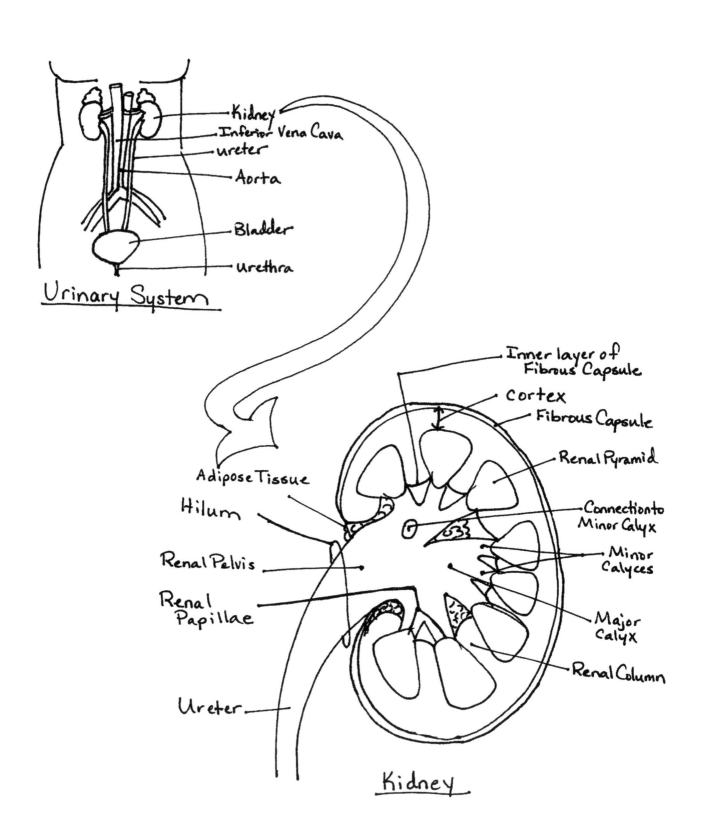

Urinary System

Kidney
Inferior Vena Cava
Ureter
Aorta
Bladder
Urethra

Inner layer of
Fibrous Capsule
Cortex
Fibrous Capsule
Renal Pyramid
Connection to
Minor Calyx
Minor
Calyces
Major
Calyx
Renal Column

Adipose Tissue
Hilum
Renal Pelvis
Renal
Papillae
Ureter

Kidney

The Nephron

Kidneys help filter the blood right? How? The kidneys are filled with microscopic tubular structures called <u>nephrons</u>. Each nephron is made of a <u>renal tubule</u> and <u>renal corpuscle</u>. The renal corpuscle is made of a <u>glomerulus</u>, which is a knot of capillaries, and a <u>Bowman's capsule</u>. I kinda think the Bowman's capsule looks a bit like a fishbowl on its side. The renal tubule is made of the <u>proximal convoluted tubule or PCT, the distal convoluted tubule or DCT and the loop of Henle</u>. In summary, blood will push into the Bowman's capsule by way of an afferent arteriole to the glomerulus and will leave the glomerulus through the efferent arteriole. The blood will then flow into the <u>peritubular capillaries</u> which surround the renal tubule and then will be off to the venous system. Filtration takes place in the renal corpuscle. Blood pressure will push water and dissolved solutes out of the glomerular capillaries and into the Bowman's capsule. We call this fluid <u>filtrate</u>. Filtrate is similar to blood plasma without the proteins. The filtrate will then enter the renal tubule which will absorb back into the body all of the useful organic nutrients, 90 percent of the water and then secrete into the tubule all wastes that did not already enter the filtrate in the glomerulus. Once the filtrate enters the tubule it is called <u>tubular fluid</u> and gradually changes along the length of the tubule eventually converting to urine. This tubular fluid enters the <u>collecting system</u> from the nephron. A collecting system is a series of tubes that carries tubular fluid away from the nephron. <u>Collecting ducts</u> receive this fluid from many nephrons. The collecting duct will empty into a <u>papillary duct</u> that will drain into a minor calyx. Approximately 85 percent of all nephrons are <u>cortical nephrons</u> which are located almost entirely within the cortex of the kidney. Their loops of Henle are short. Around 15 percent of nephrons are <u>juxtamedullary</u>. They have long loops of Henle that extend deep into the medulla.

Now let's break urine formation down in steps!

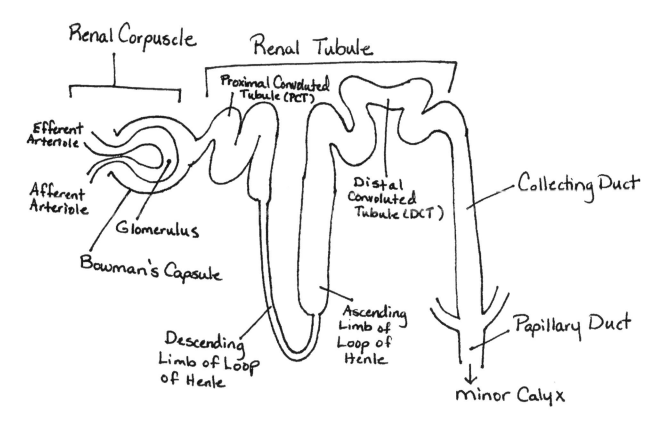

Renal Corpuscle

The lining of the Bowman's capsule is simple squamous epithelium. The visceral epithelium covers the glomerulus and is made of large cells with feet called <u>podocytes</u>. Weird huh? They are way awesome! Their feet are called <u>pedicels</u>. Things that flow out of the blood at the glomerulus must be small enough to fit between the feet or <u>filtration slits</u>. They act as filters for the blood. So you would think it was weird to find blood in your urine right? You should! Urine should not contain lots of blood! How can we filter the blood and squeeze out filtrate that contains all wastes but no blood cells? The podocytes is how! So follow this analogy…say you are boiling pasta…the ingredients are the pasta (representing blood cells) and the water (representing plasma). They are all boiling together in the pot (like how the plasma and blood cells are together in blood). When it comes time to eat you need to separate the pasta from the water so you use a colander or strainer (which represents the podocytes and their filtration slits). You put it in the sink and dump the contents of the pot, pasta and water in. What do you hope will come out of the strainer/colander? Water! The water represents plasma. What should stay in the strainer/colander? The pasta, which represents the blood cells. This is how the podocytes and filtration slits work! So if we find blood in the urine…your strainer could be broken!

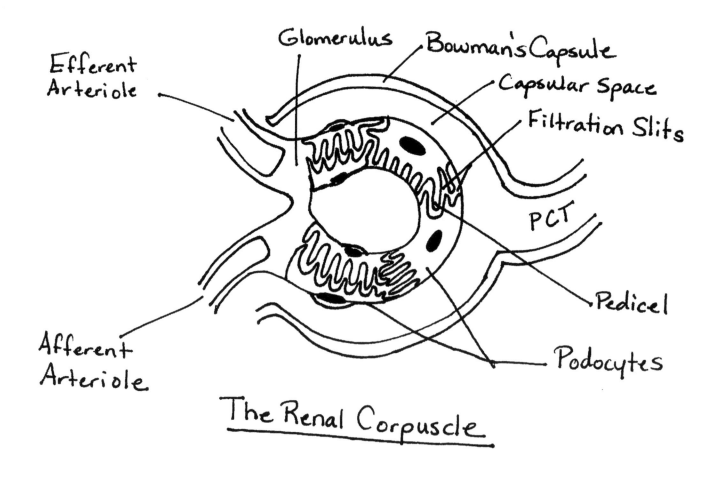

The Renal Corpuscle

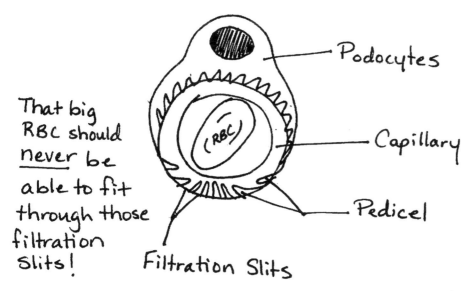

That big RBC should never be able to fit through those filtration slits!

Podocytes

Capillary

Pedicel

Filtration Slits

Zoomed In View of Capillary In Glomerulus Covered By Podocyte

During filtration, blood pressure forces water and solutes through the filtration slits into the Bowman's capsule space. The larger solutes like plasma proteins do not pass through. This is a wonderful process but the only downside is that it also lets good stuff like glucose, fatty acids, amino acids and vitamins move into the filtrate! We do not want to urinate those things out! It is up to the PCT to fix that for us!

The Proximal Convoluted Tubule or PCT

The lining of the PCT is simple cuboidal epithelia whose apical surfaces have microvilli. These cells will reabsorb (take back into the body or peritubular fluid that surrounds the nephron) organic nutrients, ions, and water. Let's be more specific, it will reabsorb: glucose, amino acids, vitamins, sodium, potassium, calcium, magnesium, phosphate, bicarbonate, water, and chloride. Reabsorption is the primary function of the PCT.

The Loop of Henle

The thick segments of the loop of Henle are lined with cuboidal epithelium and the thin are lined with squamous epithelium. The descending limb is permeable to water. The ascending limb actively and passively removes sodium and chloride ions from the tubular fluid.

The Distal Convoluted Tubule or DCT

There are no microvilli on the epithelia lining the DCT. The DCT will actively secrete (take from peritubular fluid and put into tubular fluid) toxins, drugs, ions and acids. It will also reabsorb sodium, calcium from the tubular fluid and put it back into the peritubular fluid along with water.

The Collecting System

The DCT drains into the collecting system. Individual nephrons drain into a collecting duct, several collecting ducts merge into a papillary duct which empties into a minor calyx. Two main cell types are found in the collecting duct: principal cells and intercalated cells. Intercalated cells are cuboidal cells with microvilli. Alpha-intercalated cells and beta-intercalated cells make up the population of intercalated cells. Alpha-intercalated cells secrete hydrogen ions and reabsorb bicarbonate ions, beta-intercalated cells secrete bicarbonate ions and reabsorb hydrogen ions. Principal cells are cuboidal cells that reabsorb water and secrete potassium. Together these guys help regulate the acid-base balance in the blood.

Urine Formation

Remember how we said that the act of making urine will maintain the blood's homeostasis—a blood filtration process? The goal is for us to make a urine that will excrete our metabolic wastes. These wastes are urea, creatinine and uric acid. The most abundant of these wastes is urea which is a product of the breakdown of amino acids. Skeletal muscle tissue generates creatinine from the breakdown of creatine phosphate which plays a role in muscle contraction. Finally your body produces uric acid, which is a waste formed during the recycling of nitrogenous bases from RNA molecules. These wastes are dissolved in the bloodstream and can only be eliminated when dissolved in urine.

When urine is formed, it is formed by three processes: filtration, reabsorption and secretion. Filtration occurs when blood pressure forces water and solutes through the filtration slits into the Bowman's capsule. Once the filtrate is produced it moves into the renal tubule. Reabsorption is the removal of water and solutes from the filtrate. They are moved across the epithelium of the nephron and into the peritubular fluid outside of the nephron. This process will involve simple diffusion or travel through carrier proteins in the epithelium. These reabsorbed substances eventually reenter the blood. Secretion is the movement of solutes from the peritubular fluid across the tubular epithelium into the tubular fluid. These are things we WOULD like to urinate out.

Review of transport—there are four major types of carrier-mediated transport: facilitated diffusion, active transport, cotransport and countertransport. Recall that facilitated diffusion is when a carrier protein transports a molecule across the plasma membrane without using any energy. It will move according to the concentration gradient for the ion involved. In other words, things will always flow from a high to a low concentration. Active transport is driven by ATP. Because the process is powered with energy, things can move against the concentration gradient. In co-transport, two ions/molecules or both can move across the membrane while bound to a carrier protein. Countertransport is similar to cotransport except that the two transported ions are moved in opposite directions. All of these carrier-mediated processes share features that are important to understanding kidney function. Specific substrates bind to a carrier protein that will facilitate its movement across the membrane. This movement can be active or passive. Carrier proteins usually work in one direction only. In facilitated diffusion, the concentration gradient of the substance being transported will determine the direction it will move. In active transport, cotransport and countertransport, the location of the carrier protein will determine whether a substance is reabsorbed or secreted. The distribution of carrier proteins can vary among portions of the cell surface. Transport between tubular and peritubular fluid will involve the material entering the cell at the apical surface and then leaving the cell at its basolateral surface to finally enter the peritubular fluid. The apical surface of a cell could contain, along the PCT, carrier proteins that bring amino acid, glucose and other nutrients by cotransport. Whereas the basolateral surface of the same area of the PCT may contain carrier proteins that move those nutrients out of the cell by facilitated diffusion. Carrier proteins, like enzymes can become saturated. Meaning that if more and more substrate concentration builds up to be moved across the membrane at this protein, it will not work faster. This concentration maximum is called the T_m or transport maximum.

So back to urine formation! Remember that to produce the filtrate, fluids are pushed through filtration slits into the Bowman's capsule space. This filtrate contains dissolved ions and small organic molecules. The glomerular filtration rate or GFR is the amount of filtrate the kidneys produce each minute. Filtration has to happen! If not, the wastes will build up in the blood, which can become dangerous! Filtration depends on blood flow to the glomerulus. The GFR is regulated by the hormones of the renin-angiotensin-aldosterone system. Renin is released by the juxtaglomerular apparatus or JGA (a patch of cells near the renal corpuscle). The triggers to release renin are a decrease in blood pressure at the glomerulus because of a decrease in blood volume or a blockage, stimulation of the JGA by the sympathetic nervous system, or a decrease in the osmotic concentration of the tubular fluid.

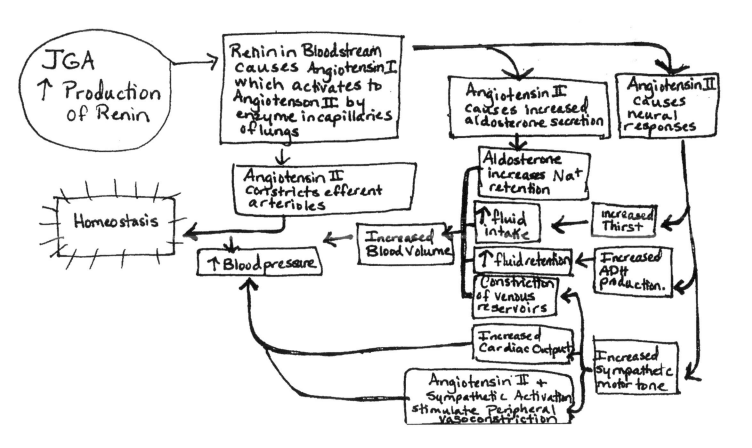

Sympathetic activation has a direct effect on the GFR. It will produce a powerful vasoconstriction (squeezing) of the afferent arterioles which will decrease the GFR and slow down filtrate production.

Okay, so once filtrate is made, on to reabsorption and secretion! Reabsorption will recover useful materials that have entered the filtrate. Secretion will get rid of wastes, toxins, and other solutes we don't want. The cells of the PCT will reabsorb 60-70% of the filtrate that was produced in the renal corpuscle. As we noted previously the reabsorption in the PCT will include 99% of glucose, amino acids and other organic nutrients. The PCT will actively transport ions like sodium, potassium, bicarbonate, magnesium, phosphate and sulfate. Water will also be reabsorbed.

The loop of Henle will reabsorb about half of the remaining water in the tubular fluid as well as two thirds of the remaining sodium and chloride. The thin descending limb and the thick ascending limb are very close together. The exchange between the two is called <u>countercurrent multiplication</u>. Here's an overview: sodium and chloride ions are pumped actively out of the thick ascending limb and into the peritubular fluid. This will dilute the tubular fluid. The pumping action increases the osmotic concentration in the peritubular fluid around the thin descending limb. This will create a concentration difference between the tubular fluid and peritubular fluid in the renal medulla. The concentration difference results in an osmotic flow of water out of the thin descending limb into the peritubular fluid. This will result in the solute concentration increasing in the thin descending limb. The arrival of the super concentrated solution in the thick ascending limb will speed the transport of sodium and chloride ions out of the loop into the peritubular fluid. This process is a way to concentrate or dilute urine.

Once the tubular fluid has entered the DCT the tubular cells will actively transport sodium and chloride out of the tubular fluid and into the peritubular fluid. Some cells will pump sodium out in exchange for potassium. The hormone aldosterone will control the sodium channels and ion pumps. It can start synthesis of sodium channels and pumps in membranes along the DCT and collecting ducts. Potassium and hydrogen secretion rates will increase or decrease in response to changes in their concentrations in peritubular fluid at any given time. The collecting ducts receive tubular fluid from many nephrons and carry it towards minor calyx. <u>Antidiuretic hormone or ADH</u> controls the permeability of the collecting system and DCT to water. We'll revisit that shortly. The collecting system reabsorbs sodium, bicarbonate and urea. The collecting system helps to control the pH of body fluids through the secretion of hydrogen and bicarbonate ions. If the pH of the peritubular fluid decreases, carrier proteins pump hydrogen ions into the tubular fluid and reabsorb bicarbonate ions that help bring us to normal pH. If the pH of the peritubular fluid rises the collecting system secretes bicarbonate ions and pumps hydrogen ions into the peritubular fluid.

Urine volume and osmotic concentration will be regulated through the control of water reabsorption through osmosis along the PCT and descending limb of the loop of Henle. The actual volume of water lost in urine is dependent on how much remaining water in the tubular fluid, after the obligatory water reabsorption that has occurred, is reabsorbed along the DCT and collecting system. These segments are impermeable to water except in the presence of ADH. This hormone causes special water channels to be inserted into the apical plasma membranes which will dramatically increase the rate of water movement back into the body. This would result in small amounts of very concentrated urine. Without ADH, water is not reabsorbed in these segments, so all the water reaching the DCT is lost in urine. This would result in large amounts of dilute urine.

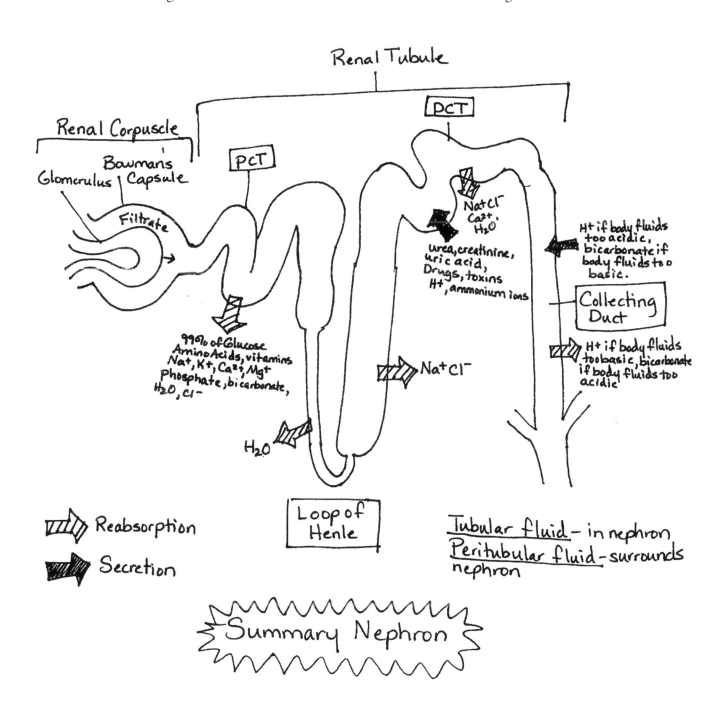

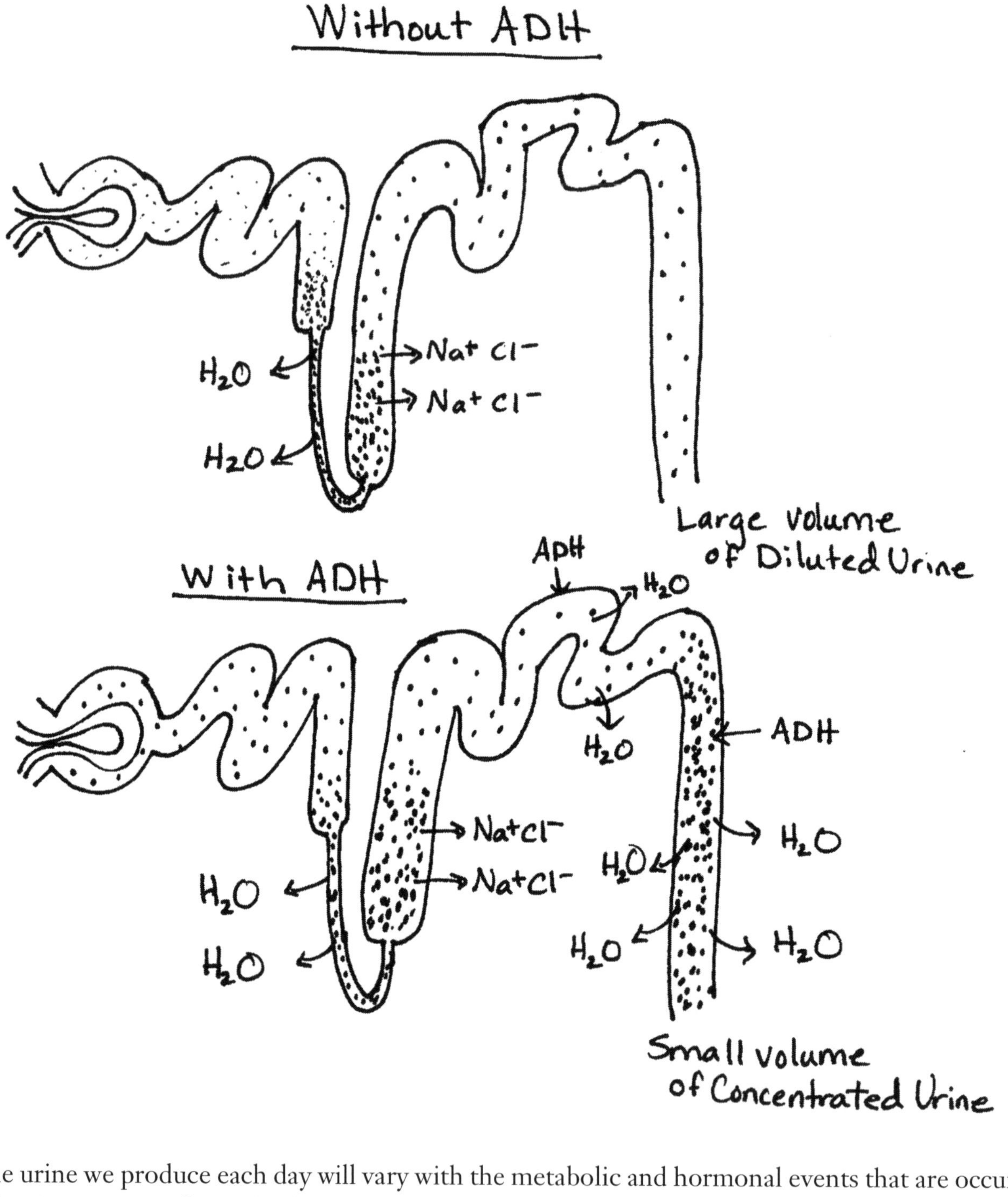

Without ADH

With ADH

ADH

H_2O

Large volume of Diluted Urine

$Na^+ Cl^-$

$Na^+ Cl^-$

H_2O

H_2O

H_2O

ADH

$Na^+ Cl^-$

$Na^+ Cl^-$

H_2O

H_2O

H_2O

H_2O

H_2O

H_2O

Small volume of Concentrated Urine

The urine we produce each day will vary with the metabolic and hormonal events that are occurring. What is in urine reflects the filtration, reabsorption and secretion of the nephrons. Normal urine is clear-ish and sterile. Its yellow color comes from the pigment urobilin. The odor of it is from the evaporation of small molecules like ammonia.

Once the urine has been created, it will enter the renal pelvis. It is now up to the ureters, bladder and urethra to aid in eliminating it. The ureters are muscular tubes that extend from the kidneys to the bladder. The ureters penetrate the posterior wall of the bladder. They open into the bladder through ureteral openings. The ureters are muscular and lined with a stretchy transitional epithelium. Peristalsis will move the urine towards the bladder. The bladder is a hollow organ for the storage of urine before elimination. Tough ligaments anchor the bladder to the pelvic and pubic bones. The lining of the bladder is full of folds like the stomach called rugae so that is able to stretch. There is a region called the trigone which is much like a funnel that channels urine into the urethra when the bladder contracts. At the base of the trigone is an internal urethral sphincter. This provides involuntary control over the discharge of urine. The muscularis externa layer of the bladder contains a detrusor muscle which is very powerful. When it is time to go it squishes the bladder and ejects urine into the urethra. The urethra transports urine to the outside of the body. In males the urethra is shared with the reproductive system and will also expel ejaculate. It attaches to the bladder and extends through to the tip of the penis. In females, the urethra is very short and is used only for urination. It is not shared with the reproductive system. In both sexes, a circular band of skeletal muscle forms the external urethral sphincter. This sphincter acts as a valve. The external urethral sphincter is voluntary and must be relaxed to allow micturition or urination.

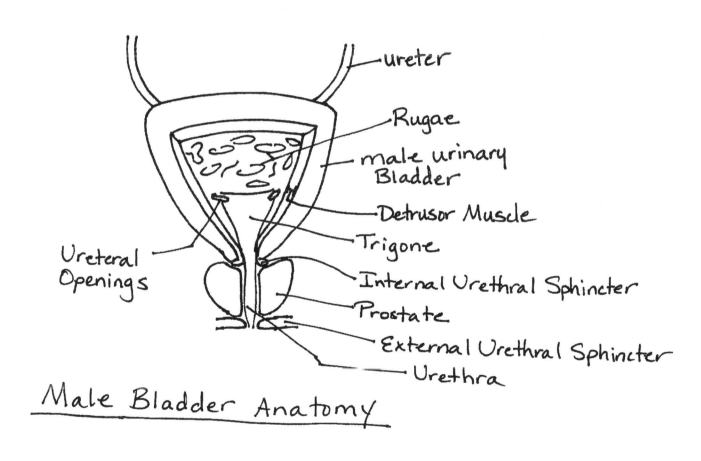

Male Bladder Anatomy

Micturition Reflex

As the bladder fills with urine, stretch receptors in the bladder wall are stimulated. Afferent fibers in the pelvic nerves will deliver impulses to the spinal cord. This will stimulate interneurons to relay these sensations to the thalamus and to the cerebral cortex giving you awareness that you gotta go! You may then relax the external urethral sphincter, which will relax the internal urethral sphincter and urination happens!

Micturition Reflex

- Stretch Receptors in the Bladder are Stimulated.

- Pelvic nerves carry impulses to the spinal cord.

- Interneurons relay sensations to the thalamus and then to cerebral cortex.

- You are now aware of the pressure in your bladder.

- You can relax the external urethral sphincter and urinate.

CHAPTER 25

Reproductive System

The reproductive system is kind of a big deal! It helps ensure the continuation of our species. Its job is to make, store, care for and release reproductive cells called gametes. The gonads are organs that make gametes and hormones. There will be various ducts that carry these gametes for eventual release and accessory glands that will make and secrete fluids to support the process. These ducts and passageways open to the outside world.

In males, the testes are the male gonads that make sex hormones called androgens. You know one of these androgens, testosterone! The testes also produce the gametes called spermatozoa or sperm. Men produce about a half a billion EVERY SINGLE DAY. Whoa. Once these spermatozoa are mixed with glandular secretions that are collectively called semen, they are released as ejaculate.

In females the ovaries are the female gonads and they produce immature gametes called oocytes. Usually one of these is released each month. This oocyte is carried along one of two fallopian or uterine tubes which end at the uterus. If a sperm finds the oocyte, fertilization may occur, but we'll explore that more when we reach chapter 26. The short passageway that connects the uterus with the outside world is called the vagina. First let's examine the anatomy of each sex.

Male Reproductive Tract

Sperm are formed in the testes and then travel through a series of ducts before they exit the body. We'll talk about each of those and then I'll give you a nice acronym to remember that pathway. The testes are enclosed within the scrotum, which is a fleshy pouch. When a fetus forms, the testes are formed inside the body cavity near the kidneys—that's a long way from home! There are connective tissue fibers that attach the testes to a little pocket in the peritoneum that will become the scrotum. These fibers are called the gubernaculum testis. The gubernacula lock the testes in position. As the fetus lengthens the testes are pulled in position gradually because they are fixed in place. Near the end of development, hormones will cause a contraction of the gubernaculum testis and the testes move into final position.

There are two spermatic cords which stretch between the abdominopelvic cavity and the testes. Each of the two cords begins at the entrance to the inguinal canal, which is a passageway through the abdominal musculature. The spermatic cord passes through the inguinal canal into the scrotum. The cord is made of the ductus deferens, blood vessels, nerves and lymphatic vessels that are surrounded by fascia and muscle. The scrotum is divided into two chambers by a structure called the raphe. Each testicle lives in a chamber called the scrotal cavity. The tunica vaginalis is a serous membrane that lines the scrotal cavity and covers the testicle. The scrotum is made of a thin layer of skin. The dermis contains a layer of smooth muscle called the dartos muscle. The dartos muscle causes the wrinkling of the scrotal surface. Under the dermis is a layer of skeletal muscle called the cremaster muscle. Due to arousal or decreased temperature, the cremaster muscle contracts the scrotum and pull the testes closer to the body. In the case of temperature, the testes should be at a temperature of 1.1°C (2°F) lower than body temperature in order for sperm production to occur normally. The cremaster and dartos muscles work together to move the testes closer to or away from the body to help maintain testicular temperature. Under the tunica vaginalis is the tunica albuginea, a layer of connective tissue with lots of collagen. The tunica albuginea also penetrates inward to form walls called septa that divide the testicle into lobules. Enclosed in the lobules are the coiled tubes called seminiferous tubules. This is where sperm production happens! These seminiferous tubules will merge into straight tubules which interconnect to form the rete testes. The rete testis is connected to the epididymis by the efferent ductules. Scattered around the tubules are Leydig cells that make androgens of which testosterone is the most important one.

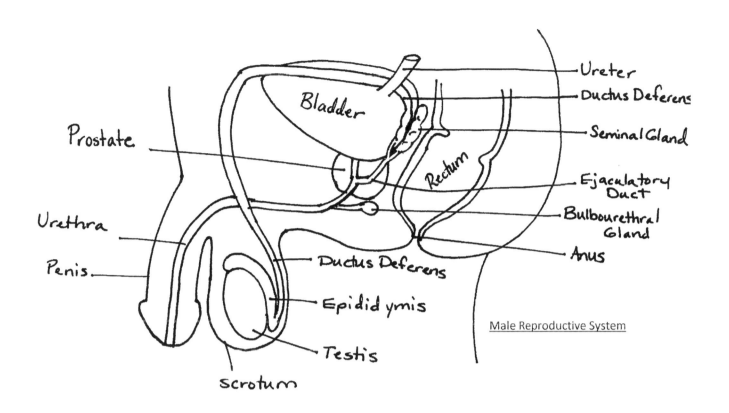

Prostate

Urethra

Penis

Bladder

Rectum

Ureter

Ductus Deferens

Seminal Gland

Ejaculatory Duct

Bulbourethral Gland

Anus

Ductus Deferens

Epididymis

Testis

Scrotum

Male Reproductive System

Zoomed In Cross-Section of Testis

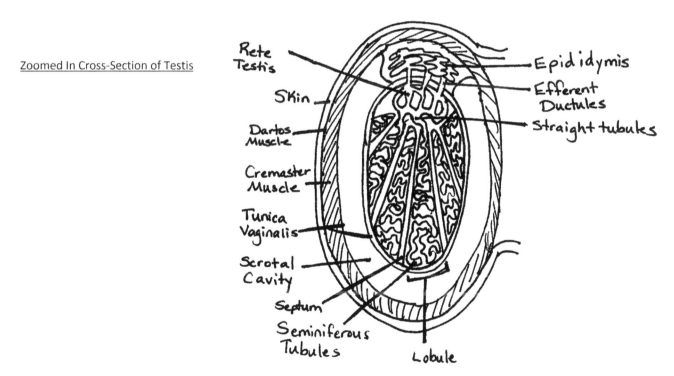

Rete Testis

Skin

Dartos Muscle

Cremaster Muscle

Tunica Vaginalis

Scrotal Cavity

Septum

Seminiferous Tubules

Epididymis

Efferent Ductules

Straight tubules

Lobule

Spermatogenesis

Spermatogenesis is the creation of sperm or spermatozoa. It happens in the walls of the seminiferous tubules. It begins in the outermost portion of the wall and as it continues the cells will be pushed towards the lumen of the tubule. Stem cells called spermatogonia will divide by mitosis to make two daughter cells. One stays to be a spermatogonium and the other will differentiate into a primary spermatocyte. Primary spermatocytes undergo meiosis—which is the process that makes gametes. Primary spermatocytes give rise to secondary spermatocytes that divide and differentiate into spermatids, which will finally differentiate into spermatozoa. The spermatozoa break free from the wall of the seminiferous tubules and enter the fluid in the lumen. Remember mitosis and meiosis? Remember how human cells that are not gametes contain 46 chromosomes? Gametes contain half that number, 23. That way when the male (23 chromosomes) and female (23 chromosomes) gamete meet, there will be 46 total chromosomes! On our way to making a new human!

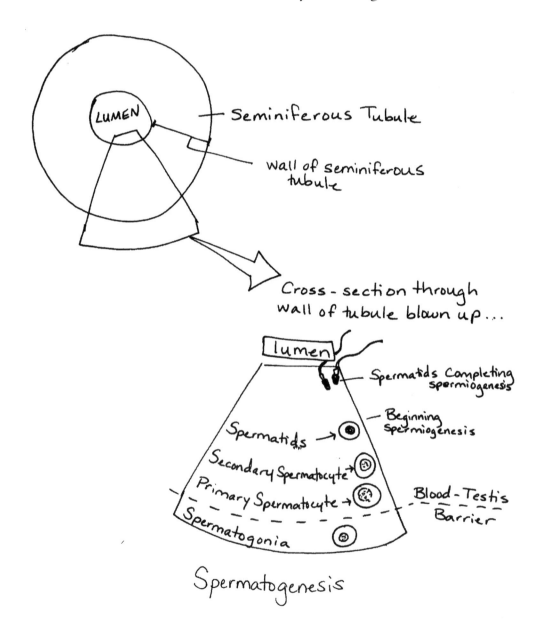

Spermatogenesis

Mitosis and Meiosis Light Review

Human somatic cells have 23 pairs of chromosomes, or a total of 46. Of that 46 total, 23 are given by mom and 23 given by dad at the time of fertilization. Mitosis is the process of somatic cell division. It results in two new daughter cells being produced, each will contain identical number and pairs of the chromosomes—still 23 pairs or 46. These are called diploid (di- double) cells.

Meiosis involves two cycles of cell division, meiosis I and II, and produces 4 new cells each containing half the number of chromosomes or 23. These cells are called haploid (single). As a cell gets ready for meiosis, the DNA replicates inside the nucleus just as it does in mitosis. As in mitosis, each chromosome now is made of two duplicate chromatids. The corresponding maternal and paternal chromosomes come together in synapsis. Synapsis involves 23 pairs of chromosomes. Each member of each pair is made of two chromatids. A matching set of four chromatids is called a tetrad. Some genetic material can be exchanged between the chromatid of a chromosome pair which is called crossing over. This increases genetic variation! In males, meiosis produces four immature gametes that are identical in size, each of these will become a sperm. In females, meiosis makes a huge oocyte and three non-functional polar bodies. If fertilization does happen, the oocyte completes meiosis II, making an ovum.

Spermiogenesis

Spermiogenesis is the last step of spermatogenesis. This is when the spermatid matures into a spermatozoon (singular for spermatozoa) or sperm. Once the spermatid becomes a spermatozoon, it will break away from the wall of the seminiferous tubule and enter the lumen of the tubule. Nurse cells are cells that help with spermatogenesis. Are you picturing them wearing little nurse hats? I was. They are going to help maintain the blood-testis barrier or BTB. The BTB will separate the seminiferous tubules from the general circulation—kinda like the blood-brain barrier! Nurse cells are stuck together by tight junctions to form a layer that divides the seminiferous tubules into an inner luminal compartment and an outer basal compartment where the spermatogonia live. The nurse cells make and regulate the fluid in the lumen of the seminiferous tubule. This fluid is filled with androgen, estrogen, amino acids and potassium. Follicle stimulating hormone FSH and testosterone cause nurse cells to activate and promote division of spermatogonia and spermatocytes. The nurse cells also promote spermiogenesis and help to move it forward by engulfing the cytoplasm the spermatid sheds to become a spermatozoon. Nurse cells secrete inhibin which is a hormone that slows the production of FSH by the pituitary. This can slow down sperm production. Each spermatozoon has a head, neck, middle piece and a tail. The head has a nucleus with 23 chromosomes and an acrosomal cap. The acrosomal cap is a compartment that contains enzymes the sperm needs to break into the egg during fertilization. The neck attaches the head to the middle piece which contains mitochondria for energy production. The sperm need ATP to move the tail. The tail is the only flagellum in the human body. It serves as a whip-like tail for the sperm to move. The mature spermatozoon lacks an endoplasmic reticulum, lysosomes, golgi, peroxisomes and other organelles. By shedding them in the process of spermiogenesis, this makes the sperm smaller and better adapted to carry the genetic material to the female gamete—should it meet one. This reduced weight will help to not slow the sperm down!

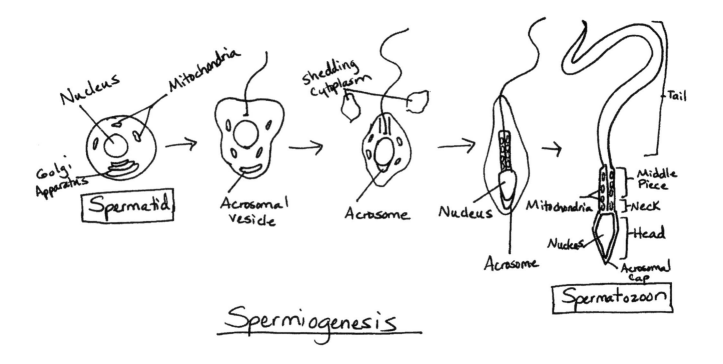

Spermiogenesis

After the sperm are formed in the seminiferous tubules, they move through the straight tubules, into the rete testis, through the efferent ductules into the <u>epididymis</u>. These sperm are physically mature but they are not ready and mature enough to fertilize an oocyte. The rest of the trip through the male reproductive tract will allow the sperm time to further mature. The overview of the path can be remembered by the acronym: SEVEN UP

S=Seminiferous tubules

E=Epididymis

V=Vas deferens (also known as ductus deferens)

E=Ejaculatory Duct

N=Nothing (space holder)

U=Urethra

P=Penis

Since the sperm have just been formed in the seminiferous tubules, they must now travel to the epididymis. At this point the sperm look ready but they cannot swim or fertilize yet. Cilia in the efferent ductules will carry these sperm into the epididymis. The epididymis has a head, body and tail region. The epididymis will check and adjust the makeup of the fluid made by the seminiferous tubules. It will also recycle damaged spermatozoa by absorbing them and releasing their products into the blood stream. It will store sperm and allow them to mature. Once they leave they will be mature but still unable to swim. To become fully mobile they must undergo capacitation. Capacitation is not widely understood yet. What is known is that the sperm will become mobile when they are mixed with secretions of the seminal glands and will only be able to fertilize when they are exposed to conditions in the female reproductive tract. The epididymis will move the sperm towards the vas or ductus deferens by fluid movement and peristalsis.

The vas or ductus deferens begins at the tail of the epididymis and moves through the inguinal canal wrapping around the back of the bladder where it enlarges to form the ampulla. Where the two ampulla join with the ducts of the seminal glands, begins the ejaculatory duct. The ejaculatory duct penetrates the prostate gland and empties into the urethra.

The urethra is a passageway that starts at the urinary bladder and ends at the tip of the penis. It has three regions: prostatic, membranous and spongy regions. It is shared by the reproductive and urinary systems

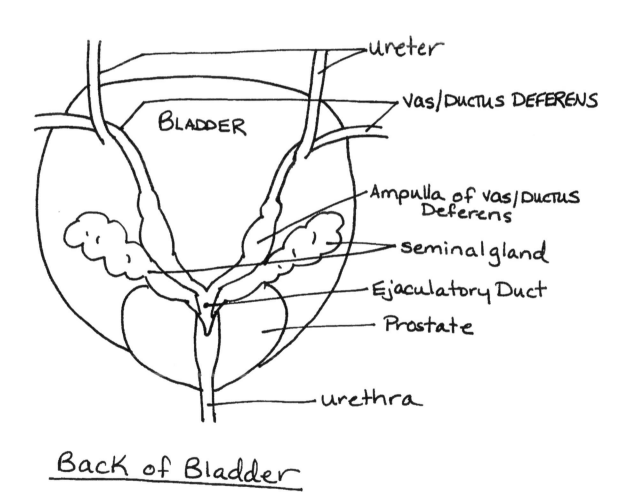

Back of Bladder

Glands

The fluid part of semen is a mixture of the secretions of the <u>seminal glands, prostate gland and bulbourethral glands.</u> They will activate sperm and give them the nutrients needed to move. They will also help to propel the sperm and fluids through the tract by peristalsis and will produce buffers that neutralize the acidity of the urethra and vaginal canal. The seminal glands secrete about 60 percent of the total volume of semen. The secretion includes fructose, which the sperm use for food to make energy and prostaglandin, which will cause smooth muscle contractions in the male and female reproductive tracts. Finally, it will contain fibrinogen which will cause the semen to thicken into a temporary clot in the vaginal canal (increasing likelihood more sperm will remain in the vaginal canal). The prostate gland is small, round and closed around the urethra under the bladder. The prostate produces prostatic fluid which is slightly acidic and makes up around 20-30 percent of the total volume of semen. The paired bulbourethral glands are located at the base of the penis. They empty a thick alkaline mucus into the urethra. This will help neutralize any urinary acids left behind in the urethra and will lubricate the tip of the penis. An average ejaculate is only 2-5 ml of semen and should contain spermatozoa (between 20-100 million spermatozoa per ml) and the seminal fluid produced by the three glands previously.

External Genitalia

The male external genitalia is the scrotum and penis. The penis is tubular and has the urethra within it. The penis is made of the <u>root, body and the glans</u>. The root is what attaches the penis to the body. The body is the moveable part of the penis and the glans is the head of the penis with the opening for urination and ejaculation. Most of the body of the penis consists of three columns of erectile tissue. The erectile tissue is a maze of vascular channels separated by walls of elastic connective tissue and smooth muscle fibers. When the penis is not erect the arterial branches in this maze are constricted and the muscular partitions are tense, this will restrict blood from entering the erectile tissue. When there is an erection, the penis hardens and elevates. When a man is relaxed, neurons release nitric oxide, which will cause the muscle of the arterial walls to relax. This will allow the vessels to dilate and for blood flow to increase so that the vascular channels in the penis become filled with blood. There are three cylinders of erectile tissue: two <u>corpora cavernosa and one corpus spongiosum</u>. Each of the corpora cavernosa surround a central artery. The corpus spongiosum surrounds the urethra.

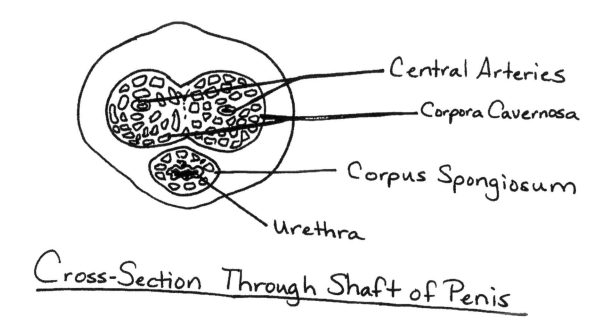

Cross-Section Through Shaft of Penis

Hormones and Male Function

Gonadotropin Releasing Hormone (GnRH) is secreted by the hypothalamus and will cause the anterior pituitary to release luteinizing hormone (LH) and follicle stimulating hormone (FSH). FSH will trigger the nurse cells of the seminiferous tubules to secrete inhibin, secrete androgen-binding protein (ABP) and promote spermatogenesis and spermiogenesis. ABP will bind androgens inside the seminiferous tubules which will stimulate the spermatids to mature.

LH will target interstitial cells of the testes to cause the secretion of testosterone and other androgens. Testosterone will maintain the sexual drive, encourage bone and muscle growth, male secondary sex characteristics and maintenance of the accessory glands and organs of the reproductive system.

Female Reproductive System

A woman's reproductive system makes sex hormones and gametes. In addition to those things a woman must be able to protect, nourish and support a developing embryo and eventually infant. The main parts of the female reproductive system are: ovaries, fallopian/uterine tubes, uterus and vagina. There are also external parts and accessory glands that will make fluids to be released into the female reproductive tract. The ovaries, fallopian tubes and uterus are closed in a mesentery called the broad ligament. The broad ligament attaches to the sides and floor of the pelvic cavity. The mesovarium is a mesentery that supports the ovary. There are two ovaries which are small, bumpy and almond shaped. They will make immature female gametes (oocytes), secrete female sex hormones and secrete inhibin which will be part of the feedback control of FSH production. The ovarian and suspensory ligaments help to hold the ovaries in place. There are blood vessels that are connected to the ovary at the ovarian hilum called the ovarian artery and ovarian vein. There is a covering on the ovary called the tunica albuginea. The ovary has an outer cortex and an inner medulla. The oocytes are made in the cortex.

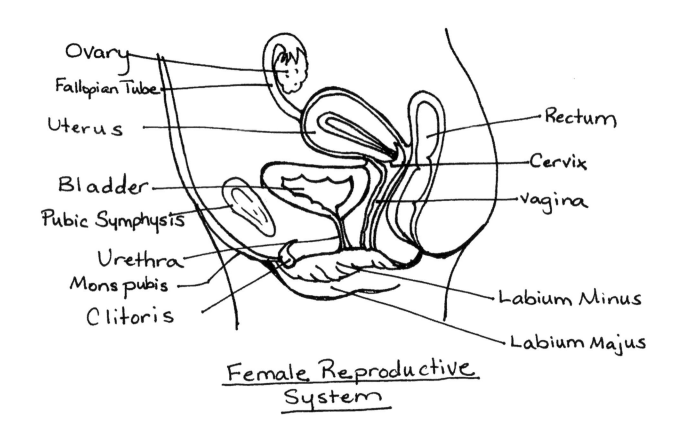

Female Reproductive
System

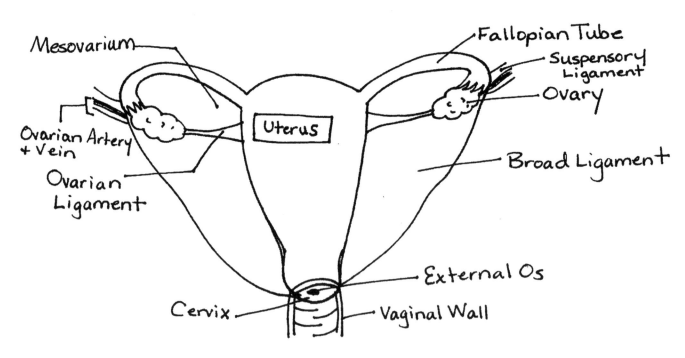

<u>Oogenesis</u>

Ovum production is called <u>oogenesis</u>. This process begins before a woman is even born, speeds up at puberty and ends in menopause. Oogenesis happens on a monthly basis and is part of the <u>ovarian cycle</u>. The female reproductive stem cells will make <u>primary oocytes</u> by the process of mitosis before birth. These cells will continue to proceed until they stop in prophase of meiosis I. They will stay in prophase of meiosis I until puberty. There are around 2 million <u>primordial follicles</u> at birth, each of those contains a primary oocyte. Primordial means—been there since the beginning of your time. Once you have reached puberty that number is less than 400,000. Let's go through the detailed steps of the ovarian cycle.

The <u>ovarian follicles</u> are structures in the cortex of the ovaries where the oocyte growth and meiosis I occur. The ovarian cycle is divided into two phases: <u>preovulatory and postovulatory</u>. In the preovulatory phase we begin with the primordial follicles in the egg nest. The primary oocytes are found in the outer portion of the ovarian cortex beside the tunica albuginea. They live in little clusters called egg nests. The primary oocyte with its follicle cells make up a primary follicle. Once someone reaches puberty, primordial follicles will be activated to begin development. The activated primordial follicle will either mature and then be released as what is called a <u>secondary oocyte</u> or degenerate (<u>atresia</u>).

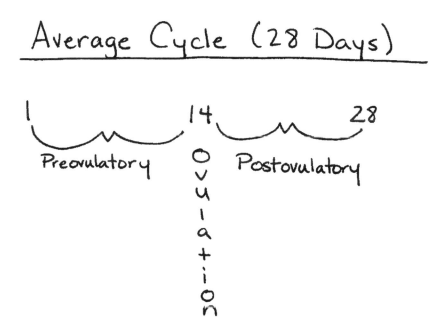

Next, follicle development begins with activation of primordial follicles. They will become <u>primary follicles</u>. The follicle cells surrounding the primary oocytes will enlarge and continue dividing, forming layers around the primary oocyte. These follicle cells are now called <u>granulosa cells</u>. The follicular cells have microvilli—remember those? The primary oocyte has microvilli on its outside. The two microvilli touch. This region is called <u>zona pellucida</u>. The large amount of microvilli in this area allow for the transfer of materials from the follicular cells to the oocyte. Wow! In other words, we are starting to baby this egg! <u>Thecal cells</u> outside the follicle form a box around the follicle and work with the granulosa cells to make estrogen.

Inside Egg Nest

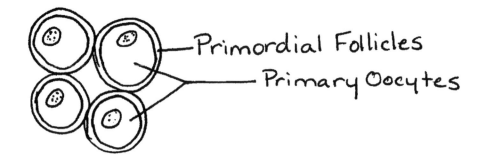

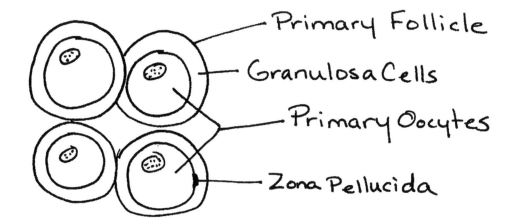

Several primordial follicles may develop into primary follicles but only a few of the primary follicles will continue to mature. The few that will move on to mature will begin to change as the wall of their follicles thickens and some of the follicular cells will produce follicular fluid. This will swell and enlarge the follicle. This larger follicle is called the <u>secondary follicle</u>. The primary oocyte will continue to grow slowly.

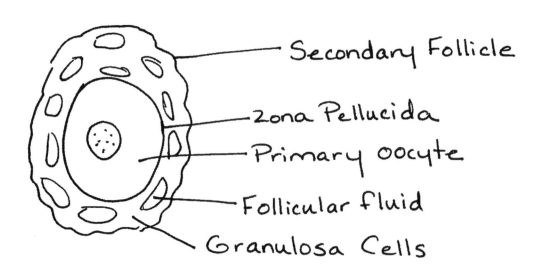

Around 8-10 days after the start of the ovarian cycle the ovaries will usually have one secondary follicle that will go on to become a <u>tertiary follicle</u>. By days 10-14 the follicle will become tertiary. This follicle is so large and so full of fluid (kind of like a cyst), it will cause a bulge on the surface of the ovary. The primary oocyte has been stuck in prophase of meiosis I. Once we near the end of the development of the tertiary follicle, there will be spike in LH (luteinizing hormone). LH will cause the oocyte to complete meiosis I. The oocyte will not split into two secondary oocytes, but instead one secondary oocyte and <u>one nonfunctional polar body</u>. When this split takes place the secondary oocyte should end up with 23 chromosomes and the nonfunctional polar body should take the extra 23. You see, up until this point the oocyte has had 46 chromosomes. Isn't that too much? YES! What would happen if a 46 chomosome'd oocyte met with a 23 chromosome'd sperm? Too much DNA! A human has 46! We need to be sure that the oocyte has 23 and the sperm has 23. That way when they meet, they make 46! Once the secondary oocyte is formed it will enter meiosis II and stop at metaphase. It will only complete meiosis if it is fertilized. So around day 14 the secondary oocyte and the granulosa cells will break away from the follicle and the granulosa cells will form a layer of protection around the oocyte called the <u>corona radiata</u>. (Like a force field!)

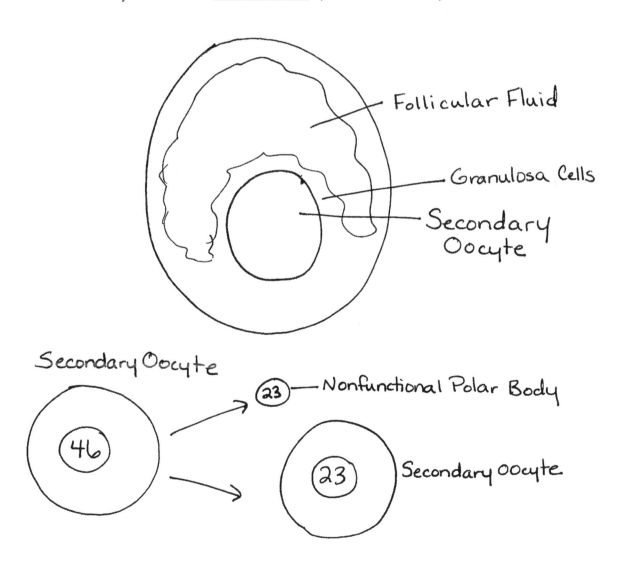

Once ovulation (release of oocyte from ovary) time is here, the tertiary follicle will release the secondary oocyte. The follicle will burst and eject the contents of the follicle including the secondary oocyte covered by the corona radiata. This sticky fluid released with the oocyte will help the corona radiata stick to the surface of the ovary. The fimbriae on the fallopian tubes will contract and move the oocyte into the fallopian tube. At this point we are at the end of the preovulatory phase!

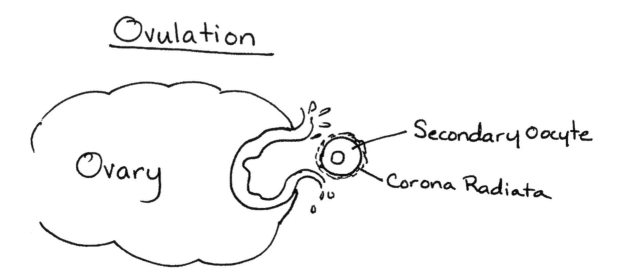

At the beginning of the postovulation phase the empty tertiary follicle changes and becomes the corpus luteum. The corpus luteum makes and releases progesterone, a hormone which will thicken the uterine lining for pregnancy. The corpus luteum will begin to break down about 12 days after ovulation—unless pregnancy happens. This will cause progesterone and estrogen levels to drop and the corpus luteum becomes a corpus albicans. This is the end of the ovarian cycle. Guess what next? We start over again! UGH!

Fallopian Tubes and Uterus

The fallopian tubes are hollow muscular tubes that have three sections or parts: the infundibulum, ampulla and isthmus. The infundibulum has little finger-like projections on it called fimbriae. The fallopian tubes are lined with ciliated epithelia. Scattered amongst this epithelia are cells called peg cells that secrete a fluid that completes capacitation of spermatozoa and gives nutrients to them. (We will discuss capacitation in the next chapter) Under the epithelia are layers of smooth muscle. The ovulated oocyte will move down the fallopian tube by way of the movement of cilia and contractions (peristalsis) of the fallopian tubes. Interestingly, the fallopian tube is filled with nutrients and lipids to nourish spermatozoa and the pre-embryo—should one form. If an oocyte isn't fertilized it will degenerate in the fallopian tube or uterus.

The uterus is a muscular organ that will protect, nourish and take away wastes for the developing embryo and fetus. When the uterus contracts it will help to push the baby out during labor. The uterus is shaped like a pear and pretty small! The body of the uterus is the largest part of it. The top portion of the uterus is rounded and is called the fundus. The cervix caps the uterus and leads to the vagina. The opening in the cervix is the <u>external os</u>. At the bottom of the <u>uterine cavity</u> is the <u>internal os</u> which leads into the <u>cervical canal</u>. The uterine wall has three layers. The outer layer is incomplete, meaning it doesn't cover the whole uterus—it is called the <u>perimetrium</u>. The middle layer is made of thick smooth muscle and is called the <u>myometrium</u>. The innermost layer is called the <u>endometrium</u> and is glandular. The glandular and vascular part of the endometrium will support the growing fetus. Estrogen will cause the glands and blood vessels of the endometrium to change with the <u>uterine cycle</u>.

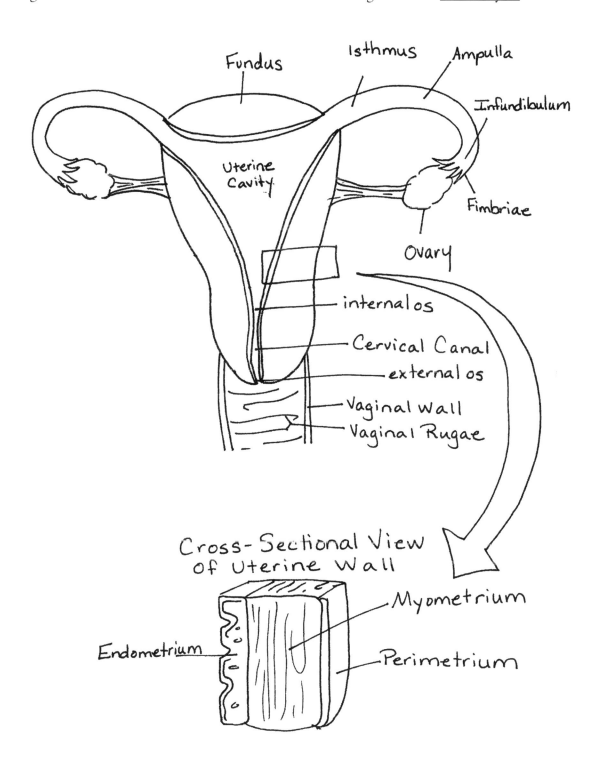

Uterine Cycle

The uterine or menstrual cycle refers to the repeating changes in the endometrial layer. The uterine cycle averages 28 days but can be between 21-35 days in healthy women. The uterine cycle has three phases: menses, proliferative and secretory. These phases are all dictated by hormones that regulate the previously talked about ovarian cycle. Menses and the proliferative phase happen during the follicular or preovulatory phase of the ovarian cycle. Secretory phase happens along the postovulatory part of the ovarian cycle. Let's examine the three phases…

Menses is when the endometrium breaks down in spots. Blood vessels that feed the endometrium will constrict and reduce the blood supply to the endometrium. What happens when you cut off blood supply to a tissue? It becomes deprived of oxygen and nutrients and will die. The broken and weakened blood vessels break and blood flows into the connective tissue. Blood cells and broken down tissue enter the uterine cavity and flow down towards the internal os, cervical canal, external os and vagina. The shedding of this tissue is gradual and repairs begin happening immediately. This can last from one to seven days.

The proliferative phase occurs after menses. This is when the epithelial cells of the uterine gland multiply and regenerate the epithelium. The uterine glands will produce glycogen rich mucous which would help a fertilized ovum to survive.

The secretory phase is when the uterine glands enlarge and secrete even more. The arteries that feed the uterine wall spiral through the tissues of the functional area of the uterus. This happens because of progesterone and estrogen from the corpus luteum. The secretory phase begins around the time of ovulation and lasts as long as the corpus luteum lasts. If pregnancy does not occur then we begin again in menses.

The uterine cycle begins at puberty with the first cycle which is called menarche. The cycles will continue until menopause which is the end of the uterine cycle. Most women go through menopause between the ages of 45-55.

The vagina is a muscular tube that begins at the cervix and ends at the exterior of the body. The vagina serves as an exit for menstrual blood, is the inferior portion of the birth canal and receives the penis during sexual intercourse. The wall of the vagina is filled with smooth muscle. The lining is kept moist by cervical glands and water that moves across the epithelium. The lumen of the vaginal canal is lined by stratified squamous epithelia which has folds called rugae. The rugae are extra tissue for expansion. The vagina has a normal, healthy population of bacteria which help to maintain an acidic environment in the vagina. This will help to deter the growth of many pathogens.

The area that holds the external genitalia is called the vulva. The vagina opens into a space called the vestibule which is surrounded by the labia minora. The greater vestibular glands are found on either side of the vagina and secrete mucous to lubricate the area. Outside the vulva is the mons pubis and the labia majora. The mons pubis is the fat pad on top of the pubic symphysis. The labia majora are folds of skin that partly cover the labia minora.

The Mammary Glands

Milk production or <u>lactation</u> takes place in the <u>mammary glands</u>. Lactation is controlled by hormones of the reproductive system and by the placenta (which we'll talk about later). The mammary gland is in the <u>pectoral fat pad</u>. In the nipple, the ducts of the mammary gland open out to the body surface. The glandular tissue of the mammary gland is made of separate lobes with <u>secretory lobules</u>. These lobules have ducts that join together to make a single <u>lactiferous duct</u>. The lactiferous duct enlarges to form a chamber called the <u>lactiferous sinus</u>. We will talk more about lactation when we get to pregnancy!

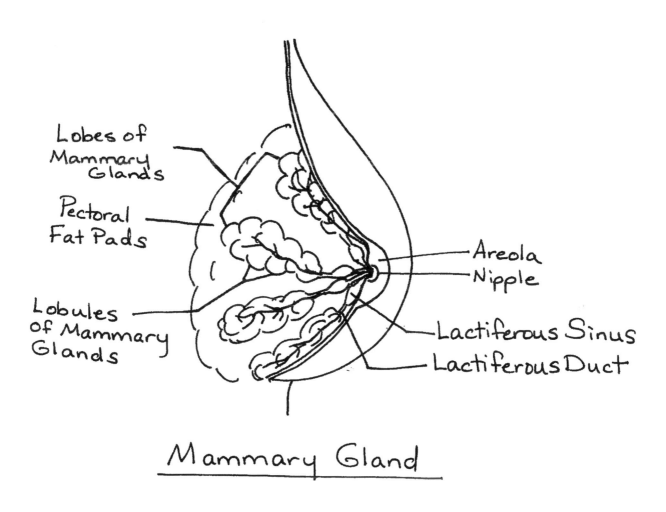

Mammary Gland

Hormones of Female Reproduction

In the preovulatory phase of the ovarian cycle (before day 10) estrogen levels are low and <u>gonadotropin releasing hormone or GnRH</u> is released in pulses around 16-24 per day. When we are at this frequency of pulses, FSH is the dominantly released hormone. Estrogen is released by forming follicles and this will inhibit LH secretion. When secondary follicles form, FSH levels go down. The follicles continue to develop and mature through the support of estrogen, FSH and LH. When we reach tertiary follicle stage, the estrogen levels go way up. This rise in estrogen causes the GnRH pulses to increase to about 36 per day. This increase will cause LH to be secreted. On around day 14 estrogen levels have peaked and the GnRH pulses are now every 30 minutes. This will cause a massive release of LH. The release of LH will trigger the completion of meiosis I by the primary oocyte, the rupture of the follicle and release or ovulation of the oocyte. Ovulation usually happens around 34-38 hours after the LH spike.

The high LH levels that start ovulation will also cause progesterone secretion and the forming of the corpus luteum. As progesterone levels go up and estrogen goes down, GnRH pulses decrease rapidly to around 1-4 times per day. This will stimulate more LH secretion to maintain the function of the corpus luteum. The corpus luteum will secrete progesterone to prepare the uterine lining for pregnancy. If no pregnancy happens, the corpus luteum breaks down and progesterone and estrogen levels drop. This will cause the endometrium to break and shed. There is no need to maintain that rich lining if no pregnancy occurs.

The primary three estrogens that circulate in the blood stream are: estradiol, estrone and estriol. Estrogens will affect many tissue and organs in the female body. It will help maintain female secondary sex characteristics (fat deposits, body hair location), increase sex drive, stimulate bone and muscle growth, maintain accessory reproductive glands and organs and help to start the repair the endometrium.

Sexual Intercourse

Sexual intercourse will allow semen into the female reproductive tract. In men, arousal occurs because of an increase in parasympathetic outflow over pelvic nerves. This will lead to erection of the penis, lubrication of the penile urethra and the head of the penis by the bulbourethral glands. Emission will occur under the sympathetic nervous system stimulation when the contractions of the vas deferens push seminal fluid and spermatozoa into the urethra inside the prostate. Ejaculation will happen when contractions in the muscles of the pelvic floor push semen toward the external urethral opening. After ejaculation, blood leaves the erectile tissue and the erection begins to go down. This is called detumescence and is also controlled by the sympathetic nervous system.

In females the sexual functions are similar. Parasympathetic activation leads to engorgement of the erectile tissue of the clitoris and increased secretion of cervical mucous glands and greater vestibular glands. This will lubricate the vaginal walls. The parasympathetic stimulation causes contraction of the muscles that control the nipples making them more sensitive.

Menopause

Menopause is the time when ovulation and menstruation stop. This is usually between the ages of 45-55. A shortage of primordial follicles is the cause of the irregular cycles leading up to menopause. As the number of the primordial follicles decreases, estrogen levels decrease and may not rise enough to trigger ovulation. Menopause is also associated by a decrease in concentrations of estrogen and progesterone and an increase in GnRH, FSH and LH. When the estrogen levels go down this can lead to a decrease in the size of the uterus and breasts and a thinning of the vaginal epithelia. The lowered amount of estrogen could also be linked to an increased rate of osteoporosis. Other side effects include hot flashes, depression and anxiety.

Male Climacteric

The time of declining reproductive function is called the <u>male climacteric</u>. Levels of testosterone began to go down between the age of 50-60. Levels of FSH and LH increase. Sperm production continues but interest in sexual activity may decline due to lowered testosterone.

Humans develop in the womb over a period of 9 months or 40 weeks. Every generation gives way to a new generation that will repeat the process. When our bodies and physiology change over time from the period of fertilization to maturity, we call that <u>development</u>. In the short time we call pregnancy, all of the cells, tissues, organs and organ systems are formed! Isn't that amazing?! When we form lots of different types of cells we call that <u>differentiation</u>. The process of differentiation is triggered by changes in genetic activity.

Development starts at <u>fertilization</u>. Fertilization is described as the time when gametes (oocyte and sperm cells) fuse. Once they fuse, there will be a series of stages of development. <u>Embryonic development</u> characterizes the changes that occur during the first two months after fertilization. <u>Fetal development</u> begins at the ninth week and continues until birth. These two phases fit into <u>prenatal development (before birth)</u>. <u>Postnatal development (after birth)</u> begins at birth. Humans go through the same developmental stages, but the difference in their genes make interesting individual characteristics.

Fertilization

The oocyte has 23 chromosomes and the sperm cell has 23 chromosomes—these are called <u>haploid gametes</u>. When the two haploid gametes fuse, this makes a <u>zygote</u>. The zygote has 46 chromosomes and is called <u>diploid</u>. The sperm cell or spermatozoon (singular for spermatozoa) delivers dad's chromosomes to the oocyte. Remember that the sperm cell has to travel and needs to be small and efficient. The oocyte must provide the mother's chromosomes, organelles, genetic programming and nourishment for the developing embryo for a week after fertilization. Due to these responsibilities the oocyte is MUCH larger than the spermatozoon. Once the spermatozoa are in the vaginal canal they are moving already. The spermatozoa can move because of coming in contact with secretions made by the seminal glands. This is the first step of <u>capacitation</u>. Capacitation is the process that causes physical changes in the sperm coating and allows receptors to be exposed on its surface. These receptors will allow it to push into the oocyte and fertilize it. The spermatozoa must also come into contact with conditions in the female's reproductive tract to fully capacitate. The mechanism behind capacitation is not fully understood at this point. The spermatozoon will fertilize an egg in the fallopian tube within a day after ovulation. The contractions of the uterus and fallopian tube cilia movement will help speed up the travel of the spermatozoa towards the secondary oocyte. Out of around 200 million spermatozoa that enter the vaginal canal in a typical ejaculate, only about 10,000 make it to the fallopian tube and only 100 make it to the isthmus of the fallopian tube. That's a lot of spermatozoa death! Everyone always says you just need one sperm cell to fertilize. That might be true, but dozens of sperm are needed to help one break into the egg for fertilization. One sperm does not have enough of the acrosomal enzymes to break through the corona radiata that surrounds the oocyte.

Once an oocyte is released in ovulation it is not functionally mature. Remember the secondary oocyte is stuck in metaphase of meiosis II? If the oocyte does not become fertilized it will disintegrate and never finish meiosis. The corona radiata is for protection around the oocyte but it also makes the process of fertilization more difficult. The sperm have to penetrate the corona radiata. The acrosomal caps contain enzymes called <u>hyaluronidase and acrosin</u>. Hyaluronidase will help to break the bonds between the cells of the corona radiata so that one sperm can penetrate the oocyte for fertilization. Many sperm cells must release these enzymes so that one sperm cell can get in. Raw deal huh? Once the sperm gets through the corona radiata it has to bind to receptors on the <u>zona pellucida</u> which surrounds the oocyte. Once a sperm binds to the receptors in the zona the acrosome ruptures and the acrosin and hyaluronidase tear a path through the zona towards the surface of the oocyte. When the sperm touches the surface, the oocyte and sperm membranes fuse triggering <u>oocyte activation</u>.

Once the sperm contacts the ooctye, the oocyte membrane will depolarize—meaning sodium will rush in and calcium will be released from the smooth endoplasmic reticulum. This will cause the <u>cortical reaction</u>. The cortical reaction will release enzymes to inactivate the sperm receptors and harden the zona. (FORCE FIELD!!) This hardening of the zona will block other sperm out. <u>Polyspermy</u> is the fertilization of one egg by more than one sperm. That would be too much DNA! The oocyte will also complete meiosis II and now the oocyte is called an <u>ovum</u>. Protein synthesis in the ovum will now be accelerated for development to begin. The nuclear material in the ovum will group up into the <u>female pronucleus</u> and the <u>male pronucleus</u>. The male and female pronuclei fuse in the process known as <u>amphimixis</u>. We now have a zygote! This zygote now has a diploid set of 46 chromosomes. The first division or cleavage of the cell is complete around 30 hours after fertilization. These two new daughter cells are called <u>blastomeres</u>.

Differentiation involves changes in the genetic activity of some cells. Information is constantly being passed between the nucleus and the cytoplasm. Chemical messages can turn on or off the activity in the nucleus. After fertilization, the zygote will divide into smaller and smaller cells that are different from each other in cytoplasmic composition which will change the genetic activity of each cell. This creates cell lines with diverse fates.

The time spent in prenatal development is called <u>gestation</u> and is divided into three <u>trimesters</u>. The <u>first trimester</u> is when the embryo and early fetus forms, as well as the beginnings of all major organ systems. The <u>second trimester</u> is when the organs and organ systems continue to develop and near completion. The <u>third trimester</u> is when the fetus grows and accumulates fat rapidly. Most of the organ systems become fully functional.

Fertilization

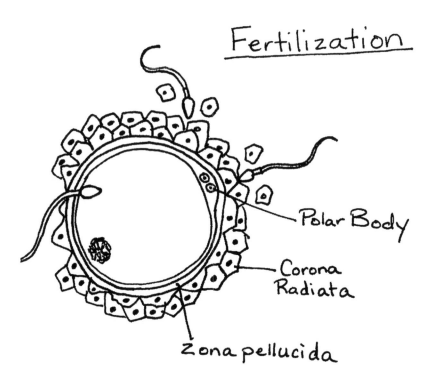

Polar Body

Corona Radiata

Zona pellucida

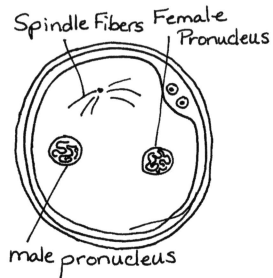

Spindle Fibers Female Pronucleus

male pronucleus

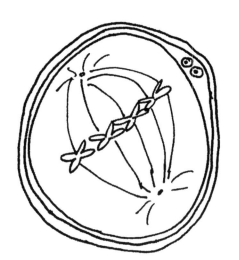

Metaphase of first cleavage division

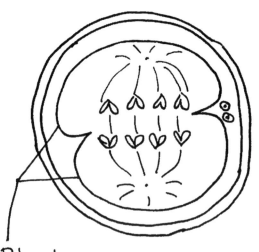

Blastomeres

The First Trimester

During the first trimester four processes must occur: <u>cleavage, implantation, placentation and embryogenesis.</u> Cleavage is when the cell divides. During cleavage the cell becomes a zygote and then a <u>pre-embryo</u> which becomes a <u>blastocyst</u>. Implantation begins when the blastocyst attaches to the endometrium of the uterus. The blastocyst burrows in. Placentation happens when blood vessels form around the blastocyst and help to form the <u>placenta</u>. The placenta is a complex organ that will allow the mother and embryo to exchange nutrients and gases without mixing blood. Embryogenesis is the formation of a viable embryo that will lay down the foundation for all major organ systems.

Remember the blastomeres? They will keep dividing. They divide as they move down the fallopian tube towards the uterus. After three days of cleavage the pre-embryo is a solid ball of cells that looks like a mulberry—this is the <u>morula</u>. Over the next two days the morula will become a <u>blastocyst</u>—a hollow ball of cells. The hollow inside is called the <u>blastocoele</u>. The outer layer of the blastocyst is called the <u>trophoblast</u> which will supply nutrients to the developing embryo. The <u>inner cell mass</u> is a cluster of cells at one end of the blastocyst. These are the cells that will become the embryo.

When the blastocyst is forming, enzymes will tear an opening in the zona so that it can be shed. This shedding is called <u>hatching</u>. The blastocyst is now exposed to fluids in the uterine cavity. It will absorb these nutrient rich fluids and enlarge. It will then attach to the endometrium and begin to implant. The inner cell mass side of the blastocyst will stick to the uterine lining about 7 days after fertilization. The trophoblast cells start dividing quickly, thickening the trophoblast. The cells closest to the inside of the blastocyst remain intact forming a layer of <u>cellular trophoblast</u>. Near the endometrium the plasma membranes between the trophoblast disappear, creating a layer of cytoplasm with lots of nuclei. This is called the <u>syncytial trophoblast</u>. The syncytial trophoblast uses hyaluronidase to dissolve a path through the uterine epithelium. The blastocyst is now implanted and has lost contact with the uterine cavity. The syncytial trophoblast will enlarge and spread. Nutrients are released by the uterine glands and are absorbed by the syncytial trophoblast. These nutrients will provide energy needed for early embryo formation. Capillary walls in the endometrium are eroded in the area and maternal blood will ooze through channels called <u>lacunae</u>. Fingerlike villi grow away from the trophoblast into the endometrium and will grow until about day 21. Blood flow will continue to speed up.

At the time of implantation the inner cell mass separates from the trophoblast creating a fluid filled sac called the <u>amniotic cavity</u>. The inner cell mass is now divided into two layers. One superficial layer faces the amniotic cavity and the second deeper layer faces the blastocoele. By day 12, a third layer of cells forms between the superficial and deep layers of the inner cell mass. The process of this cell layer formation is called <u>gastrulation</u>. The three layers are called <u>germ layers</u> and are known individually as the <u>ectoderm, mesoderm and endoderm</u>. Each of these layers will give rise to all the major organ systems of the body. AMAZING! To explore the details of what each of these layers form, please see your textbook or even better, take embryology!

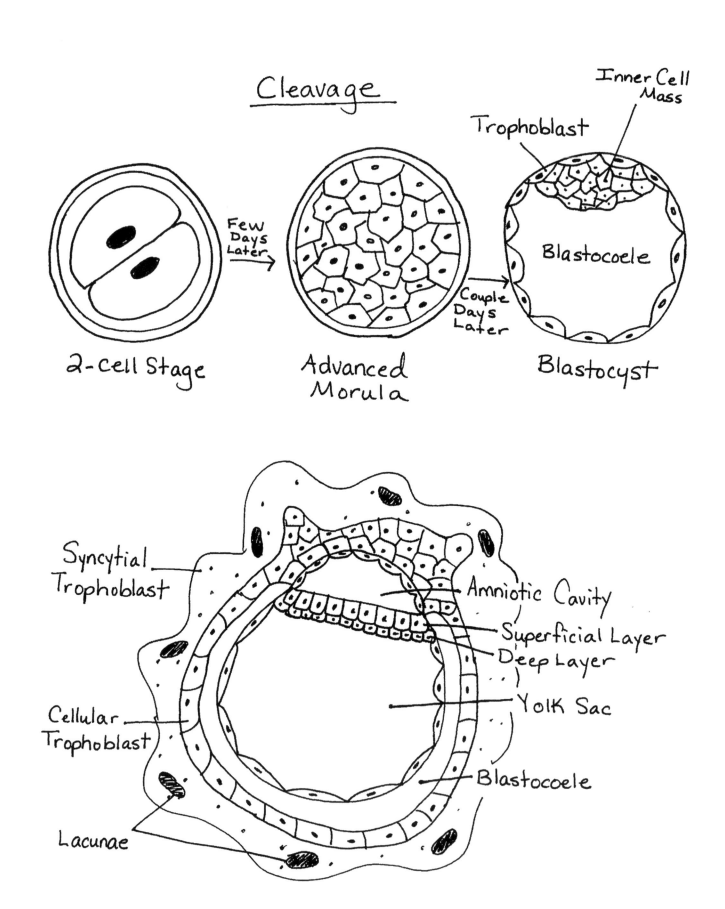

Cleavage

2-cell Stage

Few Days Later →

Advanced Morula

Couple Days Later →

Trophoblast

Inner Cell Mass

Blastocoele

Blastocyst

Syncytial Trophoblast

Cellular Trophoblast

Lacunae

Amniotic Cavity

Superficial Layer

Deep Layer

Yolk Sac

Blastocoele

The germ layers will also make four extraembryonic membranes: yolk sac, amnion, chorion and allantois. The yolk sac is formed as a layer of cells spreads around the blastocoele to form a pouch. It will be the nutrient source during early embryonic development and will give rise to blood cell formation. The amnion is formed by the spreading of ectodermal cells in the inner surface of the amniotic cavity. Amniotic fluid is made and will act as a shock absorber for the embryo. The allantois begins as part of the endoderm near the base of the yolk sac. The base of the allantois will eventually help form the urinary bladder. The chorion is critical in the maternal-embryo exchange of nutrients, gases and wastes. Diffusion alone can no longer fulfill the embryo's needs. The mesoderm spreads round the entire blastocyst separating the cellular trophoblast from the blastocoele. Blood vessels begin to develop in the mesoderm of the chorion and will form chorionic villi or fingerlike extensions that will extend into maternal tissues of the uterus. These villi will form the placenta which is where mother and fetus exchange gases and nutrients. As the chorionic villi enlarge, more maternal blood vessels erode. Maternal blood now moves through lacunae lined by the syncytial trophoblast. Chorionic blood vessels pass close by so that gases and nutrients can diffuse between the embryonic and maternal circulations. At the end of the first trimester the fetus moves farther away from the placenta but is still connected to it by the umbilical cord. Blood flows from the fetus to the placenta through the paired umbilical arteries and returns in a single umbilical vein. The chorionic villi provides a great surface area for the exchange of gases, nutrients and wastes between mom and fetus. The placenta will also produce several hormones including: human chorionic gonadotropin or hCG, placental prolactin, human placental lactogen or hPL, relaxin, progesterone and estrogen. hCG shows up in the blood soon after implantation and is a sign that a person is pregnant! This is what drug store pregnancy tests pick up on in urine. It will maintain the corpus luteum and continue the release of progesterone so that we don't lose the endometrial lining. The hCG will maintain the corpus luteum for about 3-4 months where then the placenta takes over in secreting estrogen and progesterone. hPL helps to prepare the mammary glands for milk production. It does this with the help of placental prolactin. Relaxin will be secreted by the placenta and corpus luteum and will increase the flexibility of the pubic symphysis during childbirth, help the cervix to dilate and calm the release of oxytocin to delay the onset of labor contractions. Progesterone will maintain the endometrial lining and continue the pregnancy on. The estrogen will help with labor and delivery as we shall see.

After gastrulation begins, the body of the embryo and the internal organs will start to form. This is called embryogenesis. During this time a head fold and tail fold will form. The first trimester is critical. The major beginnings of organ systems are formed but they are not functional.

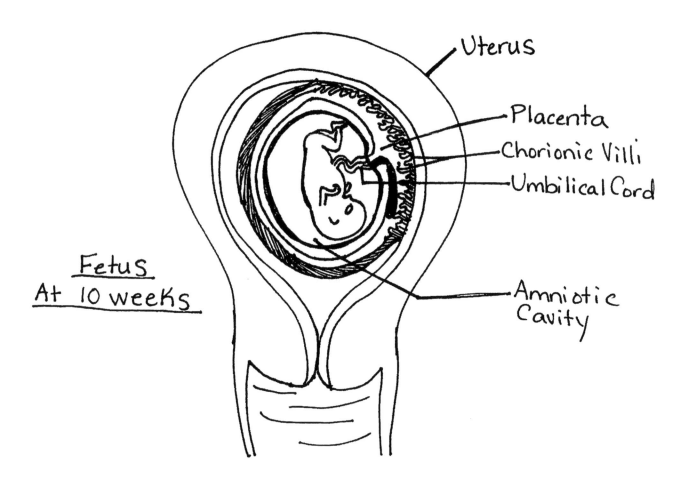

Fetus At 10 weeks

Labels: Uterus, Placenta, Chorionic Villi, Umbilical Cord, Amniotic Cavity

<u>The Second Trimester and Third Trimester</u>

Over the second trimester the fetus will grow to close to one and a half pounds. During the third trimester the organ systems becomes ready to work and perform normal functions without mom's help! The growth rate slows down but the weight gain goes up! A fetus will reach an average full-term weight of seven pounds. At the end of gestation the uterus has increased significantly in size and will push the maternal abdominal organs out of position. Because the fetus is totally dependent on the maternal systems to sustain it, the mother's body must adapt to accommodate these needs. The major changes are that the respiratory rate will increase, blood volume will increase by 50 percent, increase in nutrient uptake or appetite, glomerular filtration rate will increase by 50 percent, increase in uterine size and increase in mammary gland size and activation of milk production. At the end of gestation a typical uterus will have expanded from 7.5 cm in length to 30 cm in length. WHOA!

<u>Labor and Delivery</u>

Childbirth is the expulsion of the fetus. Contractions of the uterus begin at the top and sweep towards the cervix. As we near childbirth the contractions will increase in frequency and strength. Ouch! Labor has three phases: <u>dilation, expulsion and placental.</u>

Dilation begins as the cervix dilates and the fetus begins to move towards the cervical canal. Most women are in this stage for eight or more hours. At the start, contractions last up to half a minute and happen once every 10-30 minutes. The frequency will increase significantly. Towards the end of this stage the amniochorionic membrane will rupture ("water breaks").

Expulsion begins as the cervix, which is pushed open by the fetus, is fully dilated at 10 cm. Contractions will be SUPER strong at this point. They will last a full minute at two to three minute intervals. Expulsion will last as long as it takes to push the fetus out of the vagina. This typically lasts around 2 hours or less. If there are complications, the infant will be delivered by cesarean section. This procedure requires an incision through the abdominal wall and uterus to expose the infants head. The infant is then pulled out.

The placental stage is when final uterine contractions tear the connections between the endometrium and the placenta. The placenta will then come out.

Premature labor is when labor begins before the fetus has completed normal development. Newborns that weigh less than 14 oz at birth will not survive. Most fetuses that are born at 25-27 weeks of gestation die even with intensive care. A birth weight of 28-36 weeks is considered premature delivery. These newborns with extensive care have a good chance of survival and normal development. Babies that are face up towards the mother's sacrum during delivery, "sunny-side up," take longer to deliver and often require the use of forceps. If the legs or buttocks enter the vaginal canal first we call this breech birth. The risks are higher with babies in this position because the umbilical cord can wrap around the baby's neck or become constricted. Another risk is that the cervix may only dilate enough to accommodate the legs and buttocks but not the head. This could subject the infant to more risks.

Postnatal Stages

Neonatal period-birth to one month. The newborn must regulate its organ systems and learn to thermoregulate. The mammary glands are fully developed by the sixth month of pregnancy. The cells of the mammary gland begin to make colostrum for the first few days of the infant's life. Colostrum has more protein and less fat than breast milk. A lot of the proteins are antibodies that help the infant fight off infection until it can effectively use its own immune system. After colostrum is produced, milk production will take its place. Breast milk contains water, amino acids, proteins, lipids, sugars, salts and lysozyme. Lysozyme has antibiotic properties. This milk is made available via the milk let-down reflex.

Milk-let down reflex steps: 1) the mammary gland is stimulated by the infant sucking on the nipple, 2) these impulses move to the spinal cord and to the brain, 3) neurons are stimulated in the mom's hypothalamus, 4) hypothalamus releases oxytocin into the posterior pituitary and then enters the blood stream, 5) oxytocin causes milk ejection.

After the neonatal period of the postnatal stages is the period of <u>infancy</u> which lasts through the first year. This phase is followed by the phase of <u>childhood</u> which last from infancy to <u>adolescence</u> or puberty. Adolescence begins at puberty and ends when growth is completed. The individual is then considered physically <u>mature</u>.

Made in the USA
Columbia, SC
07 November 2020